Diverticulitis Diet Cookbook

Rose Savor

Disclaimer

Please bear in mind that the information in this book is strictly educational. The data presented here is claimed to be credible and trustworthy. The author provides no implied or explicit assurance of accuracy for specific individual instances.

It is important that you consult with a skilled practitioner, such as your doctor, before initiating any diet or lifestyle changes. The information in this book should not be used in place of expert advice or professional assistance.

The author, publisher, and distributor fully disclaim any and all liability, loss, damage, or risk suffered by anybody who relies on the information in this book, whether directly or indirectly.

All intellectual property rights are intact. The content in this book should not be copied in any way, mechanically, electronically, by photocopying, or by any other means available.

Having an invisible illness is hard to explain to someone who doesn't know it's a daily struggle feeling the pain on the inside when looking fine on the outside.

CONTENTS

A Message to the Readers

Welcome to the "Diverticulitis Diet Cookbook," where the journey to better health begins. In the pages that follow, you will find a wealth of information, practical strategies, and mouthwatering recipes designed to guide you towards managing and overcoming diverticulitis through the transformative power of a specialized diet.

As we embark on this culinary and health-focused adventure, let me share with you a remarkable success story that inspired the creation of this cookbook. One of my patients, faced with the challenges of diverticulitis, found relief and renewed well-being through the practical strategies outlined in these pages. Their journey is a testament to the efficacy of a tailored diverticulitis diet, proving that with commitment and the right guidance, individuals can take charge of their health and conquer digestive issues.

This patient's experience underscores the significance of not only understanding diverticulitis but also embracing proactive and sustainable dietary changes. Through a combination of education, personalized meal planning, and a commitment to healthier choices, they were able to regain control of their life and enjoy a more comfortable, symptom-free existence. Their success serves as a beacon of hope for everyone facing the challenges of diverticulitis, illustrating that a well-thought-out approach to nutrition can make a significant difference.

Diverticulitis is a condition that affects the digestive system, characterized by the inflammation or infection of small pouches (diverticula) that can form in the walls of the colon. This inflammation can lead to various symptoms, including abdominal pain, bloating, and changes in bowel habits. Understanding the nature of diverticulitis is crucial for developing an effective strategy to manage and alleviate its impact on daily life.

In this cookbook, we will delve into the intricacies of diverticulitis, exploring its causes, symptoms, and methods of diagnosis. Armed with this knowledge, you will be better equipped to make informed decisions about your health, paving the way for a more proactive and targeted approach to your dietary choices.

One of the cornerstones of managing diverticulitis is adopting a specialized diet that supports digestive health and minimizes the risk of flare-ups. This cookbook is crafted with precision to provide you with practical guidelines and delicious recipes tailored to the unique needs of individuals grappling with diverticulitis.

A diverticulitis-friendly diet involves a thoughtful selection of foods, emphasizing high-fiber options while avoiding certain triggers that can exacerbate symptoms. As we explore the importance of this dietary approach, you'll discover not only what to eat but also gain insights into meal planning, cooking techniques, and strategies for maintaining a balanced and enjoyable diet.

So, whether you are newly diagnosed or seeking to enhance your existing diverticulitis management plan, this cookbook is your companion on the path to digestive wellness. Let's embark on this journey together, armed with knowledge, inspiration, and the tools to savor a life free from the constraints of diverticulitis.

"I don't deserve this award, but I have diverticulitis and I don't deserve it either."

Understanding Diverticulitis

Diverticulitis is a condition that affects the gastrointestinal tract, specifically the colon, and understanding its nuances is crucial for anyone grappling with its challenges. The term "diverticulitis" refers to the inflammation or infection of small pouches, known as diverticula, which can form in the walls of the colon. These pouches are generally harmless when they first develop, but when they become infected or inflamed, they can lead to a range of uncomfortable symptoms and complications.

Causes and Risk Factors

To comprehend diverticulitis, it's essential to explore its origins. The primary cause of diverticulitis is the formation of diverticula, which are small, bulging pouches that can develop in weak spots of the colon wall. These pouches are thought to result from increased pressure on the intestinal walls, often due to a combination of factors such as age, a low-fiber diet, and a sedentary lifestyle.

Aging plays a significant role in the development of diverticulitis, as the walls of the colon naturally weaken over time. A diet low in fiber can also contribute, as it may lead to constipation and increased pressure during bowel movements. Lack of physical activity further compounds these issues, emphasizing the importance of a holistic approach to digestive health.

Symptoms and Diagnosis

Recognizing the symptoms of diverticulitis is pivotal for early intervention and effective management. Common symptoms include abdominal pain, particularly in the lower left side, bloating, changes in bowel habits, and fever. In severe cases, complications such as abscesses, perforations, or fistulas can occur, necessitating immediate medical attention.

Diagnosis typically involves a combination of medical history review, physical examination, and diagnostic tests. Imaging studies, such as CT scans, are often employed to visualize the extent of inflammation and assess the severity of the condition. A thorough understanding of the symptoms and diagnostic processes empowers individuals to seek timely medical assistance and make informed decisions about their treatment.

Impact on Daily Life

Diverticulitis is not merely a medical condition; it profoundly influences daily life. The unpredictability of symptoms can lead to discomfort, inconvenience, and a sense of loss of control. Individuals with diverticulitis may find themselves navigating dietary restrictions, altering social plans, and grappling with the emotional toll of chronic illness.

Moreover, the impact extends beyond the physical realm, affecting mental and emotional well-being. Coping with the uncertainties of diverticulitis requires resilience, support, and a comprehensive understanding of the condition's multifaceted nature.

Management and Treatment Approaches

Understanding diverticulitis is the foundation for effective management and treatment. While milder cases may be addressed through dietary changes, including increased fiber intake, severe cases may require antibiotics or, in extreme situations, surgical intervention. Lifestyle modifications, such as regular exercise and stress management, also play a pivotal role in preventing flare-ups and promoting overall digestive health.

In conclusion, a comprehensive understanding of diverticulitis encompasses its causes, symptoms, impact on daily life, and various approaches to management. Armed with this knowledge, individuals can engage in proactive measures to enhance their quality of life and work towards a future free from the constraints of this gastrointestinal condition.

"It takes some balls to live life to the fullest."

The Importance of Diet in Diverticulitis

Diet plays a pivotal role in the management and prevention of diverticulitis, a condition characterized by the inflammation or infection of small pouches in the colon. Understanding the relationship between diet and diverticulitis is essential for individuals seeking to alleviate symptoms, prevent flare-ups, and cultivate overall digestive health.

High-Fiber Diet: A Cornerstone of Diverticulitis Management

A high-fiber diet is widely regarded as a cornerstone in the management of diverticulitis. Fiber, found in fruits, vegetables, whole grains, and legumes, adds bulk to the stool, softens it, and facilitates regular bowel movements. These effects are particularly crucial for diverticulitis patients, as a diet rich in fiber can help prevent constipation and reduce the pressure on the colon walls, thereby lowering the risk of diverticula formation and inflammation.

Foods to Embrace and Avoid

Understanding which foods to embrace and which to avoid is key to tailoring a diet that supports diverticulitis management. High-fiber foods, such as broccoli, apples, and beans, are generally recommended. On the flip side, certain foods may exacerbate symptoms and should be consumed in moderation or avoided altogether. These may include nuts, seeds, and popcorn, as their small, hard particles can potentially get lodged in the diverticula, leading to irritation and inflammation.

Hydration and its Impact on Digestive Health

Hydration is often an overlooked yet integral aspect of a diverticulitis-friendly diet. Ample water intake is crucial for maintaining soft and pliable stools, preventing constipation, and promoting overall digestive health. Individuals with diverticulitis should prioritize staying well-hydrated, as dehydration can contribute to the hardening of stools, making bowel movements more challenging and potentially triggering flare-ups.

Meal Planning Strategies for Diverticulitis Patients

Strategic meal planning is a valuable tool for individuals managing diverticulitis. Small, frequent meals that include a balance of fiber-rich foods and lean proteins can help maintain stable blood sugar levels and reduce the strain on the digestive system. Portion control is also essential to avoid overloading the digestive tract, promoting more comfortable and efficient digestion.

The Role of Probiotics in Digestive Wellness

Probiotics, beneficial bacteria that support a healthy gut microbiome, have gained recognition for their potential role in managing digestive conditions, including diverticulitis. These microorganisms contribute to a balanced gut environment, aiding in digestion and immune function. Incorporating probiotic-rich foods, such as yogurt and fermented vegetables, or considering supplements under the guidance of a healthcare professional, can be part of a holistic approach to digestive wellness.

Lifestyle Factors: Exercise and Stress Management

Diet is only one component of a comprehensive approach to diverticulitis management. Regular exercise and stress management also play integral roles in promoting digestive wellness. Exercise stimulates bowel function, helping to regulate bowel movements, while stress reduction techniques, such as mindfulness and relaxation exercises, can contribute to a healthier gut environment.

The importance of diet in diverticulitis cannot be overstated. A well-balanced, high-fiber diet, coupled with hydration, strategic meal planning, and attention to lifestyle factors, forms a powerful strategy for managing symptoms and preventing flare-ups. As individuals navigate their journey towards digestive wellness, a personalized and informed approach to dietary choices becomes a guiding force in achieving lasting relief and an improved quality of life.

Foundations of a Diverticulitis-Friendly Diet

A diverticulitis-friendly diet is not merely a list of restrictions; it is a carefully crafted blueprint that empowers individuals to manage and overcome the challenges posed by this gastrointestinal condition. By understanding the foundations of such a diet, individuals can lay the groundwork for improved digestive health, reduced symptoms, and an enhanced overall quality of life.

High-Fiber Foods: The Cornerstone of Nutritional Strategy

At the heart of a diverticulitis-friendly diet lies a commitment to high-fiber foods. Fiber is an indigestible substance found in plant-based foods that passes through the digestive system relatively intact, adding bulk to the stool and promoting regular bowel movements. For individuals with diverticulitis, a high-fiber diet serves as a crucial preventive measure, reducing the risk of diverticula formation and inflammation.

The spectrum of high-fiber foods includes fruits like apples, pears, and berries; vegetables such as broccoli, carrots, and leafy greens; whole grains like oats, brown rice, and quinoa; and legumes, including beans and lentils. By incorporating a variety of these fiber-rich options into daily meals, individuals can support digestive function and minimize the likelihood of constipation—a common concern for those with diverticulitis.

Importance of Hydration: Softening the Path to Digestive Health

Hydration is a fundamental aspect of a diverticulitis-friendly diet. Water plays a crucial role in softening stools, facilitating their movement through the digestive tract, and preventing constipation. Inadequate water intake can contribute to hardened stools, exacerbating symptoms and potentially triggering diverticulitis flare-ups.

In addition to water, herbal teas, and broths can contribute to overall hydration. It's essential for individuals to pay attention to their fluid intake, especially in times of increased fiber consumption, as fiber absorbs water in the digestive tract, necessitating additional fluid to maintain optimal digestive function.

Balanced Nutrient Intake: Nourishing the Body, Supporting Healing

A diverticulitis-friendly diet is not solely about fiber; it encompasses a balanced intake of essential nutrients. Proteins, found in lean meats, poultry, fish, eggs, and plant-based sources like tofu and legumes, play a vital role in tissue repair and overall health. Healthy fats, derived from sources such as avocados, nuts, and olive oil, contribute to satiety and provide essential fatty acids with anti-inflammatory properties.

Incorporating a variety of nutrient-dense foods ensures that individuals receive a broad spectrum of vitamins and minerals, promoting overall well-being and supporting the body's healing processes. A balanced nutrient intake is especially crucial for diverticulitis patients, as it helps maintain strength, energy levels, and resilience in the face of digestive challenges.

Moderation and Avoidance: Tailoring the Diet to Individual Needs

While high-fiber foods form the foundation of a diverticulitis-friendly diet, it's equally important to exercise in moderation and, in some cases, avoid specific foods. Nuts, seeds, and popcorn, for instance, contain small, hard particles that may pose a risk of irritation and inflammation within diverticula. While these foods can be enjoyed in moderation by some individuals, those prone to diverticulitis flare-ups may find it beneficial to limit or avoid them.

Similarly, processed foods, high in refined sugars and low in nutritional value, can contribute to inflammation and digestive discomfort. Customizing the diet to individual tolerances and preferences is a key aspect of crafting a sustainable and effective diverticulitis management plan.

Meal Planning Strategies: Practical Approaches for Everyday Success

Effective meal planning is a practical strategy that transforms the principles of a diverticulitis-friendly diet into everyday habits. Breaking meals into smaller, more frequent portions can ease the digestive burden, preventing overloading of the gastrointestinal tract. Incorporating a mix of fiber-rich foods, proteins, and healthy fats into each meal ensures a well-rounded and satisfying diet.

Additionally, meal planning involves mindful choices when dining out or ordering food. Individuals with diverticulitis can communicate their dietary needs to restaurants, opting for menu items that align with their nutritional requirements. Planning ahead and having diverticulitis-friendly snacks on hand can also prevent impulsive choices that may exacerbate symptoms.

In conclusion, the foundations of a diverticulitis-friendly diet rest on the principles of high-fiber foods, hydration, balanced nutrient intake, moderation and avoidance, and practical meal planning. By embracing these elements, individuals can cultivate a diet that not only addresses the specific challenges of diverticulitis but also promotes sustained digestive wellness and an improved quality of life.

"Failure will never overtake me if my determination to succeed is strong enough."

Lifestyle Changes for Long-Term Wellness in Diverticulitis Management

Achieving long-term wellness for individuals with diverticulitis involves more than just dietary modifications; it necessitates a holistic approach that encompasses various lifestyle changes. These adjustments aim to reduce symptoms, prevent flare-ups, and enhance overall well-being. By adopting the following lifestyle changes, individuals can take proactive steps toward sustained digestive health.

Regular Physical Activity

Exercise is a powerful contributor to overall wellness and digestive health. Engaging in regular physical activity helps stimulate bowel function, promoting more efficient and regular bowel movements. This is particularly beneficial for individuals with diverticulitis, as it can prevent constipation—a common trigger for diverticulitis flare-ups.

Various forms of exercise, such as brisk walking, jogging, cycling, and yoga, can be tailored to individual preferences and fitness levels. Incorporating moderate exercise into the daily routine not only supports digestive function but also contributes to weight management and overall cardiovascular health.

Stress Management Techniques

Stress has been linked to exacerbating symptoms in many digestive conditions, including diverticulitis. Adopting stress management techniques is crucial for individuals seeking long-term wellness. Practices such as meditation, deep breathing exercises, and mindfulness can help reduce stress levels and contribute to a more harmonious gut environment.

It's essential for individuals to identify stress triggers in their lives and develop coping strategies that work for them. Whether it's through relaxation techniques, hobbies, or counseling, managing stress effectively can significantly impact the frequency and severity of diverticulitis symptoms.

Adequate Hydration

Hydration is a fundamental aspect of digestive health, and it plays a critical role in diverticulitis management. Ample water intake softens stools, facilitates their movement through the digestive tract, and helps prevent constipation—a potential precursor to diverticulitis flare-ups.

Individuals should aim to drink an adequate amount of water throughout the day, adjusting their fluid intake based on factors such as diet, climate, and physical activity level. Hydration also extends beyond water, including herbal teas and broths that contribute to overall fluid balance.

Regular Medical Check-ups

Routine medical check-ups are essential for individuals with diverticulitis, allowing healthcare professionals to monitor the condition and make necessary adjustments to the management plan. Regular follow-ups provide an opportunity to discuss any changes in symptoms, assess the effectiveness of dietary and lifestyle interventions, and address emerging concerns.

Healthcare providers may recommend imaging studies or other diagnostic tests to evaluate the status of diverticula and assess the overall health of the digestive system. These check-ups serve as a proactive measure to catch potential issues early and ensure a personalized and effective long-term management plan.

Consistent Medication Adherence: Staying on Course with Treatment

For some individuals with diverticulitis, medication may be part of the long-term management plan. Whether it's antibiotics during flare-ups or medications to address specific symptoms, consistent adherence to the prescribed treatment is crucial for maintaining symptom control and preventing complications.

Individuals should communicate openly with their healthcare providers about any challenges or concerns regarding medication adherence. Adjustments to the medication regimen may be made based on the individual's response and evolving health needs.

Breakfast

Quinoa Breakfast Bowl with Berries

Start your day with a nutrient-packed Quinoa Breakfast Bowl featuring the wholesome goodness of quinoa and a burst of flavorful berries.

Total Time: 20 minutes
Servings: 2

Ingredients:
- 1 cup cooked quinoa
- 1 cup mixed berries (strawberries, blueberries, raspberries)
- 1/4 cup chopped nuts (almonds, walnuts)
- 2 tablespoons honey
- 1/2 teaspoon vanilla extract
- 1/2 cup Greek yogurt

Directions:
1. In a bowl, combine the cooked quinoa, mixed berries, chopped nuts, honey, and vanilla extract.
2. Mix well until all ingredients are evenly distributed.
3. Divide the quinoa mixture into serving bowls.
4. Top each bowl with a generous dollop of Greek yogurt.
5. Drizzle with an extra swirl of honey if desired.
6. Serve immediately and enjoy this delicious and protein-packed breakfast!

Nutritional Information (per serving):
- Calories: 320
- Protein: 12g
- Carbohydrates: 50g
- Fat: 8g
- Fiber: 7g

Greek Yogurt Parfait with Almond Granola

Indulge in a Greek Yogurt Parfait that combines the creaminess of Greek yogurt with the crunch of almond granola and the sweetness of fresh fruits.

Total Time: 15 minutes
Servings: 2

Ingredients:
- 1 cup Greek yogurt
- 1/2 cup almond granola
- 1/2 cup mixed berries (strawberries, blueberries)
- 1 tablespoon honey
- 1/4 teaspoon cinnamon

Directions:
1. In serving glasses or bowls, layer Greek yogurt, almond granola, and mixed berries.
2. Drizzle honey over each layer and sprinkle with a touch of cinnamon.
3. Repeat the layers until the glass is filled.
4. Finish with a dollop of Greek yogurt, a sprinkle of granola, and a few berries on top.
5. Serve immediately, savoring the delightful textures and flavors.

Nutritional Information (per serving):
- Calories: 280
- Protein: 15g
- Carbohydrates: 35g
- Fat: 10g
- Fiber: 6g

Oatmeal Pancakes with Blueberry Compote

Transform your breakfast with these hearty Oatmeal Pancakes topped with a luscious blueberry compote for a perfect blend of comfort and flavor.

Total Time: 30 minutes
Servings: 4

Ingredients:

For the Pancakes:
- 1 cup old-fashioned oats
- 1 cup milk (dairy or plant-based)
- 1 ripe banana
- 1 egg
- 1 teaspoon baking powder
- 1/2 teaspoon cinnamon
- Pinch of salt

For the Blueberry Compote:
- 1 cup fresh or frozen blueberries
- 2 tablespoons maple syrup
- 1 tablespoon lemon juice

Directions:

For the Pancakes:
1. In a blender, combine oats, milk, banana, egg, baking powder, cinnamon, and a pinch of salt.
2. Blend until smooth to create the pancake batter.
3. Heat a non-stick skillet over medium heat and pour 1/4 cup of batter per pancake.
4. Cook until bubbles form on the surface, then flip and cook the other side.
5. Repeat until all batter is used.

For the Blueberry Compote:
1. In a saucepan, combine blueberries, maple syrup, and lemon juice.
2. Simmer over low heat until the blueberries burst and the mixture thickens.

Serve the pancakes topped with blueberry compote and enjoy!

Nutritional Information (per serving):
- Calories: 240
- Protein: 8g
- Carbohydrates: 42g
- Fat: 5g
- Fiber: 5g

Scrambled Eggs with Spinach and Feta

Elevate your morning routine with these Scrambled Eggs featuring the vibrant flavors of spinach and feta, creating a protein-packed and satisfying breakfast.

Total Time: 15 minutes
Servings: 2

Ingredients:
- 4 large eggs
- 1 cup fresh spinach, chopped
- 1/4 cup crumbled feta cheese
- Salt and pepper to taste
- 1 tablespoon olive oil

Directions:
1. In a bowl, whisk the eggs until well beaten.
2. Heat olive oil in a non-stick skillet over medium heat.
3. Add chopped spinach and sauté until wilted.
4. Pour the beaten eggs over the spinach, stirring gently.
5. As the eggs begin to set, add crumbled feta cheese and continue stirring until fully cooked.
6. Season with salt and pepper to taste.
7. Serve immediately, savoring the creamy texture and savory flavors.

Nutritional Information (per serving):
- Calories: 280
- Protein: 18g
- Carbohydrates: 3g
- Fat: 22g
- Fiber: 1g

Chia Seed Pudding with Sliced Banana

Dive into a delightful Chia Seed Pudding, a nutritious and energy-boosting breakfast option topped with fresh sliced bananas for a naturally sweet touch.

Total Time: 4 hours (includes chilling time)
Servings: 2

Ingredients:
- 1/4 cup chia seeds
- 1 cup almond milk
- 1 tablespoon maple syrup
- 1/2 teaspoon vanilla extract
- 1 ripe banana, sliced

Directions:
1. In a bowl, combine chia seeds, almond milk, maple syrup, and vanilla extract.
2. Whisk the mixture thoroughly and let it sit for 5 minutes.
3. Whisk again to avoid clumping, then cover and refrigerate for at least 4 hours or overnight.
4. Before serving, stir the pudding to achieve a smooth consistency.
5. Spoon the chia pudding into serving bowls and top with sliced bananas.
6. Drizzle with a bit of additional maple syrup if desired.
7. Enjoy the creamy, nutrient-packed goodness of this Chia Seed Pudding!

Nutritional Information (per serving):
- Calories: 180
- Protein: 4g
- Carbohydrates: 30g
- Fat: 6g
- Fiber: 9g

Smoothie Bowl with Kale and Pineapple

Energize your morning with a refreshing Smoothie Bowl featuring the vibrant flavors of kale and pineapple, creating a nutrient-packed and delicious start to your day.

Total Time: 10 minutes
Servings: 2

Ingredients:
- 2 cups kale leaves, stemmed and chopped
- 1 cup frozen pineapple chunks
- 1 banana
- 1/2 cup Greek yogurt
- 1 tablespoon chia seeds
- 1/2 cup almond milk
- Toppings: sliced kiwi, granola, shredded coconut

Directions:

1. In a blender, combine kale, frozen pineapple, banana, Greek yogurt, chia seeds, and almond milk.
2. Blend until smooth and creamy.
3. Pour the smoothie into bowls and top with sliced kiwi, granola, and shredded coconut.
4. Serve immediately, enjoying the vibrant colors and flavors of this nutritious breakfast.

Nutritional Information (per serving):

- Calories: 250
- Protein: 10g
- Carbohydrates: 45g
- Fat: 6g
- Fiber: 10g

Buckwheat Waffles with Mixed Berries

Treat yourself to a wholesome breakfast with Buckwheat Waffles, a delightful combination of nutty buckwheat flavor topped with a medley of mixed berries.

Total Time: 25 minutes
Servings: 4

Ingredients:

- 1 cup buckwheat flour
- 1 cup whole wheat flour
- 1 tablespoon baking powder
- 1/2 teaspoon cinnamon
- 2 eggs
- 1 3/4 cups almond milk
- 2 tablespoons melted coconut oil
- Toppings: mixed berries, maple syrup

Directions:

1. Preheat your waffle iron according to the manufacturer's instructions.
2. In a large bowl, whisk together buckwheat flour, whole wheat flour, baking powder, and cinnamon.
3. In a separate bowl, beat the eggs and add almond milk and melted coconut oil.
4. Pour the wet ingredients into the dry ingredients, stirring until just combined.
5. Ladle the batter onto the preheated waffle iron and cook until golden brown.
6. Serve the waffles with a generous topping of mixed berries and a drizzle of maple syrup.

Nutritional Information (per serving):
- Calories: 320
- Protein: 10g
- Carbohydrates: 45g
- Fat: 12g
- Fiber: 8g

Avocado Toast with Poached Egg

Elevate your morning with Avocado Toast topped with a perfectly poached egg, creating a breakfast that's not only delicious but also rich in healthy fats and protein.

Total Time: 15 minutes
Servings: 2

Ingredients:
- 2 slices whole grain bread
- 1 ripe avocado, mashed
- 2 large eggs
- Salt and pepper to taste
- Optional toppings: red pepper flakes, microgreens

Directions:
1. Toast the slices of whole grain bread until golden brown.
2. Spread mashed avocado evenly over each slice.
3. In a pot of simmering water, poach the eggs until whites are set but yolks remain runny.
4. Carefully place one poached egg on each avocado toast.
5. Sprinkle with salt and pepper to taste and add optional toppings like red pepper flakes or microgreens.
6. Serve immediately, savoring the creamy avocado and perfectly poached egg.

Nutritional Information (per serving):
- Calories: 280
- Protein: 12g
- Carbohydrates: 20g
- Fat: 18g
- Fiber: 8g

Cottage Cheese and Fruit Salad

Enjoy a light and protein-packed breakfast with Cottage Cheese and Fruit Salad, a refreshing combination of creamy cottage cheese and a variety of fresh fruits.

Total Time: 10 minutes
Servings: 2

Ingredients:
- 1 cup low-fat cottage cheese
- 1 cup mixed fresh fruits (strawberries, pineapple, grapes, kiwi)
- 2 tablespoons honey
- 1/4 cup chopped nuts (almonds, walnuts)

Directions:
1. In a bowl, spoon the cottage cheese.
2. Add mixed fresh fruits on top.
3. Drizzle honey over the fruit and cottage cheese.
4. Sprinkle with chopped nuts for added crunch.
5. Gently toss the ingredients together.
6. Serve immediately, relishing the combination of creamy, sweet, and nutty flavors.

Nutritional Information (per serving):
- Calories: 280
- Protein: 18g
- Carbohydrates: 30g
- Fat: 10g
- Fiber: 5g

Sweet Potato Hash with Turkey Sausage

Spice up your breakfast with Sweet Potato Hash featuring flavorful turkey sausage, creating a hearty and satisfying morning meal.

Total Time: 30 minutes
Servings: 4

Ingredients:
- 2 medium sweet potatoes, peeled and diced
- 1/2 pound turkey sausage, crumbled

- 1 red bell pepper, diced
- 1 onion, finely chopped
- 2 cloves garlic, minced
- 1 teaspoon smoked paprika
- Salt and pepper to taste
- 2 tablespoons olive oil
- Optional toppings: chopped fresh parsley, poached eggs

Directions:
1. Heat olive oil in a large skillet over medium heat.
2. Add diced sweet potatoes and cook until tender and slightly crispy.
3. Push sweet potatoes to one side and add turkey sausage to the skillet, cooking until browned.
4. Stir in diced bell pepper, chopped onion, and minced garlic.
5. Season with smoked paprika, salt, and pepper to taste.
6. Continue cooking until vegetables are tender and flavors are well combined.
7. Serve the Sweet Potato Hash on plates, adding optional toppings like chopped fresh parsley or poached eggs.

Nutritional Information (per serving):
- Calories: 320
- Protein: 15g
- Carbohydrates: 30g
- Fat: 18g
- Fiber: 5g

Almond Flour Banana Muffins

These Almond Flour Banana Muffins are a delightful and gluten-free way to start your day. Packed with the natural sweetness of ripe bananas and the nutty goodness of almond flour, they are a wholesome treat for breakfast.

Total Time: 30 minutes
Servings: 12 muffins

Ingredients:
- 2 cups almond flour
- 1/2 teaspoon baking soda
- 1/4 teaspoon salt
- 3 ripe bananas, mashed

- 3 large eggs
- 1/4 cup coconut oil, melted
- 1 teaspoon vanilla extract
- Optional: chopped nuts or dark chocolate chips for topping

Directions:
1. Preheat the oven to 350°F (175°C) and line a muffin tin with paper liners.
2. In a large bowl, whisk together almond flour, baking soda, and salt.
3. In a separate bowl, mix mashed bananas, eggs, melted coconut oil, and vanilla extract.
4. Combine the wet and dry ingredients until just mixed.
5. Spoon the batter into muffin cups, filling each about two-thirds full.
6. Optional: Top each muffin with chopped nuts or dark chocolate chips.
7. Bake for 20-25 minutes or until a toothpick comes out clean.
8. Allow the muffins to cool before serving.

Nutritional Information (per muffin):
- Calories: 180
- Protein: 6g
- Carbohydrates: 11g
- Fat: 14g
- Fiber: 3g

Salmon and Asparagus Omelet

Indulge in a protein-packed breakfast with this Salmon and Asparagus Omelet. Filled with omega-3-rich salmon and nutrient-dense asparagus, this omelet is a delicious way to kick-start your day.

Total Time: 15 minutes
Servings: 2

Ingredients:
- 4 large eggs
- 1/2 cup cooked salmon, flaked
- 1/2 cup asparagus, chopped
- 1/4 cup feta cheese, crumbled
- Salt and pepper to taste
- Fresh dill for garnish (optional)
- 1 tablespoon olive oil

Directions:

1. In a bowl, whisk the eggs and season with salt and pepper.
2. Heat olive oil in a non-stick skillet over medium heat.
3. Add chopped asparagus and cook until tender.
4. Pour the whisked eggs into the skillet, swirling to spread evenly.
5. Sprinkle flaked salmon and crumbled feta cheese over one-half of the omelet.
6. Once the edges set, carefully fold the omelet in half.
7. Cook for an additional minute until the cheese melts.
8. Garnish with fresh dill if desired and serve hot.

Nutritional Information (per serving):

- Calories: 320
- Protein: 24g
- Carbohydrates: 4g
- Fat: 23g
- Fiber: 2g

Apple Cinnamon Quinoa Porridge

Warm up your morning with a comforting bowl of Apple Cinnamon Quinoa Porridge. This gluten-free and protein-rich porridge is infused with the natural sweetness of apples and the warmth of cinnamon.

Total Time: 25 minutes
Servings: 4

Ingredients:

- 1 cup quinoa, rinsed
- 2 cups almond milk
- 2 apples, peeled and diced
- 1 teaspoon cinnamon
- 1/4 cup chopped walnuts
- 1 tablespoon maple syrup (optional)
- Pinch of salt

Directions:

1. In a saucepan, combine quinoa, almond milk, diced apples, cinnamon, and a pinch of salt.
2. Bring the mixture to a boil, then reduce heat to low and simmer for 15-20 minutes, or until quinoa is cooked.

3. Stir in chopped walnuts and maple syrup if desired.
4. Simmer for an additional 5 minutes, allowing the flavors to meld.
5. Serve the porridge warm, adjusting sweetness to taste.

Nutritional Information (per serving):
- Calories: 280
- Protein: 9g
- Carbohydrates: 46g
- Fat: 8g
- Fiber: 6g

Blueberry Almond Smoothie

Kickstart your day with the vibrant flavors of a Blueberry Almond Smoothie. Packed with antioxidants from blueberries and the nutty goodness of almonds, this smoothie is a delicious and nutritious breakfast option.

Total Time: 10 minutes
Servings: 2

Ingredients:
- 1 cup blueberries (fresh or frozen)
- 1 banana
- 1/4 cup almond butter
- 1 cup almond milk
- 1 tablespoon chia seeds
- Ice cubes (optional)
- Honey for sweetness (optional)

Directions:
1. In a blender, combine blueberries, banana, almond butter, almond milk, and chia seeds.
2. Blend until smooth and creamy.
3. Add ice cubes if a colder consistency is desired.
4. Optional: Sweeten with honey to taste.
5. Pour the smoothie into glasses and enjoy the refreshing burst of flavors.

Nutritional Information (per serving):
- Calories: 300
- Protein: 8g

- Carbohydrates: 32g
- Fat: 18g
- Fiber: 7g

Spinach and Mushroom Breakfast Wrap

Wrap up a nutritious breakfast with this Spinach and Mushroom Breakfast Wrap. Packed with leafy greens, protein-rich eggs, and savory mushrooms, this delicious wrap is perfect for a quick and satisfying morning meal.

Total Time: 15 minutes
Servings: 2

Ingredients:
- 4 large eggs, beaten
- 1 cup spinach leaves
- 1 cup mushrooms, sliced
- 1/2 cup feta cheese, crumbled
- 2 whole grain tortillas
- Salt and pepper to taste
- 1 tablespoon olive oil

Directions:
1. In a skillet, heat olive oil over medium heat.
2. Add sliced mushrooms and sauté until golden brown.
3. Add spinach leaves to the skillet and cook until wilted.
4. Pour beaten eggs over the vegetables and scramble until fully cooked.
5. Season with salt and pepper to taste.
6. Warm the whole grain tortillas in the skillet or microwave.
7. Spoon the egg and vegetable mixture onto each tortilla.
8. Sprinkle crumbled feta cheese over the top.
9. Fold the sides of the tortilla over the filling, creating a wrap.
10. Serve the Spinach and Mushroom Breakfast Wrap warm and enjoy!

Nutritional Information (per serving):
- Calories: 320
- Protein: 16g
- Carbohydrates: 22g
- Fat: 20g
- Fiber: 5g

Lunch

Grilled Chicken Salad with Mixed Greens

Enjoy a light and flavorful Grilled Chicken Salad with Mixed Greens. This salad combines tender grilled chicken with a variety of fresh greens, creating a wholesome and satisfying lunch option.

Total Time: 20 minutes
Servings: 2

Ingredients:
- 2 boneless, skinless chicken breasts
- 6 cups mixed salad greens
- 1 cup cherry tomatoes, halved
- 1 cucumber, sliced
- 1/4 cup red onion, thinly sliced
- 1/4 cup feta cheese, crumbled
- 2 tablespoons balsamic vinaigrette dressing
- Salt and pepper to taste
- Olive oil for grilling

Directions:
1. Preheat the grill or grill pan over medium-high heat.
2. Season chicken breasts with salt and pepper and brush with olive oil.
3. Grill the chicken for 6-8 minutes per side or until fully cooked.
4. In a large bowl, toss mixed greens, cherry tomatoes, cucumber, red onion, and feta cheese.
5. Slice grilled chicken and arrange on top of the salad.
6. Drizzle with balsamic vinaigrette dressing.
7. Toss the salad gently to combine all ingredients.
8. Serve the Grilled Chicken Salad immediately, savoring the combination of flavors and textures.

Nutritional Information (per serving):
- Calories: 320
- Protein: 30g
- Carbohydrates: 15g
- Fat: 16g
- Fiber: 5g

Quinoa and Black Bean Stuffed Peppers

Elevate your lunch with these Quinoa and Black Bean Stuffed Peppers. Packed with protein, fiber, and a variety of colorful vegetables, these stuffed peppers are a nutritious and satisfying meal.

Total Time: 45 minutes
Servings: 4

Ingredients:
- 4 large bell peppers, halved and seeds removed
- 1 cup quinoa, cooked
- 1 can (15 oz) black beans, drained and rinsed
- 1 cup corn kernels (fresh or frozen)
- 1 cup cherry tomatoes, diced
- 1/2 cup red onion, finely chopped
- 1 teaspoon cumin
- 1 teaspoon chili powder
- Salt and pepper to taste
- 1 cup shredded cheddar cheese
- Fresh cilantro for garnish (optional)

Directions:
1. Preheat the oven to 375°F (190°C).
2. In a large bowl, combine cooked quinoa, black beans, corn, cherry tomatoes, red onion, cumin, chili powder, salt, and pepper.
3. Stuff each bell pepper half with the quinoa and black bean mixture.
4. Top each stuffed pepper with shredded cheddar cheese.
5. Place the stuffed peppers in a baking dish and cover with aluminum foil.
6. Bake for 25-30 minutes or until the peppers are tender.
7. Remove the foil and bake for an additional 5 minutes to melt the cheese.
8. Garnish with fresh cilantro if desired and serve these Quinoa and Black Bean Stuffed Peppers hot.

Nutritional Information (per serving):
- Calories: 380
- Protein: 18g
- Carbohydrates: 55g
- Fat: 12g
- Fiber: 12g

Turkey and Avocado Wrap with Whole Grain Tortilla

Savor the flavors of a Turkey and Avocado Wrap with Whole Grain Tortilla. This wholesome and protein-packed wrap is not only delicious but also a convenient and satisfying lunch option.

Total Time: 15 minutes
Servings: 2

Ingredients:
- 4 whole grain tortillas
- 1/2 pound deli-sliced turkey
- 1 avocado, sliced
- 1 cup mixed greens
- 1/4 cup cherry tomatoes, halved
- 2 tablespoons Greek yogurt
- 1 tablespoon Dijon mustard
- Salt and pepper to taste

Directions:
1. In a small bowl, mix Greek yogurt and Dijon mustard.
2. Lay out whole grain tortillas and spread the yogurt-mustard sauce evenly.
3. Layer each tortilla with deli-sliced turkey, avocado slices, mixed greens, and cherry tomatoes.
4. Season with salt and pepper to taste.
5. Roll the tortillas into wraps, securing with toothpicks if needed.
6. Slice the wraps in half and serve these Turkey and Avocado Wraps immediately.

Nutritional Information (per serving):
- Calories: 350
- Protein: 20g
- Carbohydrates: 35g
- Fat: 15g
- Fiber: 8g

Lentil Soup with Spinach and Tomatoes

Warm up your lunch with a hearty Lentil Soup infused with spinach and tomatoes. Packed with protein and fiber, this soup is not only nutritious but also a flavorful and comforting option.

Total Time: 40 minutes
Servings: 6

Ingredients:
- 1 cup dried green lentils, rinsed
- 1 onion, diced
- 2 carrots, peeled and sliced
- 2 celery stalks, chopped
- 3 cloves garlic, minced
- 1 can (14 oz) diced tomatoes
- 4 cups vegetable broth
- 2 cups baby spinach leaves
- 1 teaspoon cumin
- 1 teaspoon paprika
- Salt and pepper to taste
- 2 tablespoons olive oil
- Fresh parsley for garnish

Directions:
1. In a large pot, heat olive oil over medium heat.
2. Add diced onion, sliced carrots, chopped celery, and minced garlic. Sauté until vegetables are softened.
3. Add dried lentils, diced tomatoes, vegetable broth, cumin, paprika, salt, and pepper.
4. Bring the soup to a boil, then reduce heat and simmer for 25-30 minutes or until lentils are tender.
5. Stir in baby spinach leaves and cook until wilted.
6. Adjust seasoning to taste and serve the Lentil Soup hot, garnished with fresh parsley.

Nutritional Information (per serving):
- Calories: 220
- Protein: 13g
- Carbohydrates: 35g
- Fat: 4g
- Fiber: 10g

Tuna Salad Lettuce Wraps

Experience a light and refreshing lunch with Tuna Salad Lettuce Wraps. These wraps are filled with a zesty tuna salad mixture, offering a protein-rich and low-carb option for a satisfying meal.

Total Time: 15 minutes
Servings: 4

Ingredients:
- 2 cans (5 oz each) tuna, drained
- 1/4 cup mayonnaise
- 1 tablespoon Dijon mustard
- 1 celery stalk, finely chopped
- 1/4 cup red onion, finely chopped
- 1 tablespoon capers, drained
- Salt and pepper to taste
- Butter lettuce leaves for wrapping
- Sliced cucumber for garnish

Directions:
1. In a bowl, combine drained tuna, mayonnaise, Dijon mustard, chopped celery, chopped red onion, and capers.
2. Mix until well combined.
3. Season with salt and pepper to taste.
4. Spoon the tuna salad onto butter lettuce leaves, creating wraps.
5. Garnish with sliced cucumber and serve these Tuna Salad Lettuce Wraps immediately.

Nutritional Information (per serving):
- Calories: 180
- Protein: 20g
- Carbohydrates: 2g
- Fat: 10g
- Fiber: 1g

Mediterranean Chickpea Salad

Delight your taste buds with the vibrant flavors of the Mediterranean Chickpea Salad. This refreshing salad is a symphony of colors and textures, featuring chickpeas, cherry tomatoes, cucumber, feta, and a zesty lemon dressing.

Total Time: 15 minutes
Servings: 4

Ingredients:
- 2 cans (15 oz each) chickpeas, drained and rinsed
- 1 cup cherry tomatoes, halved
- 1 cucumber, diced
- 1/2 red onion, finely chopped
- 1/2 cup Kalamata olives, sliced
- 1/2 cup feta cheese, crumbled
- 1/4 cup fresh parsley, chopped
- 3 tablespoons extra-virgin olive oil
- 2 tablespoons lemon juice
- Salt and pepper to taste

Directions:
1. In a large bowl, combine chickpeas, cherry tomatoes, cucumber, red onion, olives, feta, and parsley.
2. In a small bowl, whisk together olive oil, lemon juice, salt, and pepper.
3. Pour the dressing over the salad and toss gently to coat all ingredients.
4. Adjust seasoning to taste and serve this Mediterranean Chickpea Salad as a refreshing lunch option.

Nutritional Information (per serving):
- Calories: 320
- Protein: 12g
- Carbohydrates: 35g
- Fat: 16g
- Fiber: 10g

Broccoli and Cheddar Soup

Warm up your lunchtime with a comforting bowl of Broccoli and Cheddar Soup. This creamy and flavorful soup combines the goodness of broccoli with the richness of cheddar cheese for a satisfying meal.

Total Time: 30 minutes
Servings: 6

Ingredients:
- 4 cups broccoli florets
- 1 onion, diced
- 2 carrots, peeled and sliced
- 3 cups vegetable broth
- 2 cups shredded cheddar cheese
- 2 cups milk (dairy or plant-based)
- 1/4 cup all-purpose flour
- 3 tablespoons unsalted butter
- Salt and pepper to taste
- Optional: croutons for garnish

Directions:
1. In a pot, melt butter over medium heat. Add diced onion and sliced carrots, cooking until softened.
2. Stir in flour to create a roux, then slowly whisk in vegetable broth and milk.
3. Add broccoli florets to the pot and simmer until vegetables are tender.
4. Use an immersion blender to puree the soup until smooth.
5. Stir in shredded cheddar cheese until melted.
6. Season with salt and pepper to taste.
7. Serve the Broccoli and Cheddar Soup hot, garnished with croutons if desired.

Nutritional Information (per serving):
- Calories: 280
- Protein: 14g
- Carbohydrates: 18g
- Fat: 18g
- Fiber: 4g

Shrimp and Quinoa Bowl with Roasted Vegetables

Enjoy a protein-packed lunch with the Shrimp and Quinoa Bowl featuring succulent shrimp, quinoa, and a medley of roasted vegetables. This bowl is not only nutritious but also bursting with delicious flavors.

Total Time: 40 minutes
Servings: 4

Ingredients:
- 1 cup quinoa, cooked
- 1 pound shrimp, peeled and deveined
- 2 cups broccoli florets
- 1 red bell pepper, sliced
- 1 zucchini, sliced
- 2 tablespoons olive oil
- 1 teaspoon smoked paprika
- 1 teaspoon garlic powder
- Salt and pepper to taste
- Lemon wedges for serving
- Fresh parsley for garnish

Directions:
1. Preheat the oven to 400°F (200°C).
2. In a bowl, toss shrimp, broccoli, red bell pepper, and zucchini with olive oil, smoked paprika, garlic powder, salt, and pepper.
3. Spread the mixture on a baking sheet in a single layer.
4. Roast in the oven for 20-25 minutes or until shrimp is cooked and vegetables are tender.
5. In serving bowls, assemble the Shrimp and Quinoa Bowl by layering cooked quinoa and the roasted shrimp and vegetables.
6. Garnish with fresh parsley and serve with lemon wedges.

Nutritional Information (per serving):
- Calories: 350
- Protein: 25g
- Carbohydrates: 30g
- Fat: 14g
- Fiber: 5g

Zucchini Noodles with Pesto and Cherry Tomatoes

Embrace a light and flavorful lunch with Zucchini Noodles with Pesto and Cherry Tomatoes. This low-carb and gluten-free option features zucchini noodles tossed in a vibrant pesto sauce, topped with cherry tomatoes for a burst of freshness.

Total Time: 20 minutes
Servings: 2

Ingredients:
- 4 medium zucchinis, spiralized into noodles
- 1 cup cherry tomatoes, halved
- 1/2 cup fresh basil leaves
- 1/4 cup pine nuts
- 1/4 cup grated Parmesan cheese
- 2 cloves garlic
- 1/2 cup extra-virgin olive oil
- Salt and pepper to taste
- Optional: red pepper flakes for garnish

Directions:
1. In a food processor, combine fresh basil, pine nuts, Parmesan cheese, garlic, salt, and pepper.
2. While the processor is running, slowly pour in the olive oil until a smooth pesto sauce forms.
3. In a large pan, sauté zucchini noodles until just tender.
4. Toss the zucchini noodles with the pesto sauce until well coated.
5. Add cherry tomatoes and toss gently to combine.
6. Serve the Zucchini Noodles with Pesto and Cherry Tomatoes immediately, garnished with red pepper flakes if desired.

Nutritional Information (per serving):
- Calories: 280
- Protein: 6g
- Carbohydrates: 10g
- Fat: 25g
- Fiber: 3g

Brown Rice and Veggie Sushi Rolls

Dive into a lunchtime delight with Brown Rice and Veggie Sushi Rolls. These homemade rolls feature nutrient-rich brown rice, colorful vegetables, and the savory taste of seaweed, providing a satisfying and healthy lunch option.

Total Time: 30 minutes
Servings: 4 (8 rolls)

Ingredients:
- 2 cups cooked brown rice
- 4 sheets nori (seaweed)
- 1 cucumber, julienned
- 1 carrot, julienned
- 1 avocado, sliced
- 1/2 cup pickled ginger
- Soy sauce for dipping
- Wasabi and sesame seeds for garnish (optional)

Directions:
1. Place a sheet of nori on a bamboo sushi rolling mat.
2. Wet your hands and spread a thin layer of brown rice over the nori, leaving a border at the top.
3. Arrange julienned cucumber, carrot, and avocado along the bottom edge of the rice.
4. Carefully roll the nori and rice over the vegetables, using the sushi mat to shape the roll.
5. Seal the edge with a bit of water.
6. Repeat the process with the remaining nori sheets and ingredients.
7. Slice each roll into bite-sized pieces using a sharp, wet knife.
8. Serve the Brown Rice and Veggie Sushi Rolls with pickled ginger, soy sauce, and optional garnishes like wasabi and sesame seeds.

Nutritional Information (per serving):
- Calories: 240
- Protein: 5g
- Carbohydrates: 45g
- Fat: 5g

Hummus and Veggie Wrap

Elevate your lunch with the Hummus and Veggie Wrap, a delightful combination of colorful vegetables, creamy hummus, and a whole grain tortilla. This wrap is not only delicious but also a nutritious option for a satisfying midday meal.

Total Time: 15 minutes
Servings: 2

Ingredients:
- 4 whole grain tortillas
- 1 cup hummus
- 1 cucumber, julienned
- 1 bell pepper, thinly sliced
- 1 carrot, shredded
- 1/2 cup cherry tomatoes, halved
- 1/4 cup red onion, thinly sliced
- 1/2 cup mixed greens
- Salt and pepper to taste

Directions:
1. Lay out whole grain tortillas and spread a generous layer of hummus over each.
2. Evenly distribute julienned cucumber, sliced bell pepper, shredded carrot, cherry tomatoes, red onion, and mixed greens on each tortilla.
3. Season with salt and pepper to taste.
4. Roll the tortillas into wraps, securing with toothpicks if needed.
5. Slice the wraps in half and serve the Hummus and Veggie Wrap immediately.

Nutritional Information (per serving):
- Calories: 300
- Protein: 10g
- Carbohydrates: 45g
- Fat: 10g
- Fiber: 8g

Sweet Potato and Black Bean Chili

Warm up your lunch with the hearty and flavorful Sweet Potato and Black Bean Chili. This vegetarian chili is packed with protein, fiber, and the natural sweetness of sweet potatoes, creating a comforting and nutritious meal.

Total Time: 45 minutes
Servings: 6

Ingredients:
- 2 sweet potatoes, peeled and diced
- 2 cans (15 oz each) black beans, drained and rinsed
- 1 can (14 oz) diced tomatoes
- 1 onion, diced
- 2 bell peppers, diced
- 2 cloves garlic, minced
- 2 tablespoons chili powder
- 1 tablespoon cumin
- 1 teaspoon smoked paprika
- Salt and pepper to taste
- 4 cups vegetable broth
- Olive oil for cooking
- Optional toppings: avocado, cilantro, shredded cheese

Directions:
1. In a large pot, sauté diced onion and bell peppers in olive oil until softened.
2. Add minced garlic, chili powder, cumin, smoked paprika, salt, and pepper. Stir to coat the vegetables.
3. Add diced sweet potatoes, black beans, diced tomatoes, and vegetable broth to the pot.
4. Bring the chili to a boil, then reduce heat and simmer for 30-35 minutes or until sweet potatoes are tender.
5. Adjust seasoning to taste.
6. Serve the Sweet Potato and Black Bean Chili hot, garnished with avocado, cilantro, and shredded cheese if desired.

Nutritional Information (per serving):
- Calories: 280
- Protein: 10g
- Carbohydrates: 55g
- Fat: 2g
- Fiber: 14g

Chicken and Vegetable Stir-Fry

Enjoy a quick and flavorful lunch with the Chicken and Vegetable Stir-Fry. This stir-fry features tender chicken, crisp vegetables, and a savory sauce, creating a balanced and delicious meal.

Total Time: 25 minutes
Servings: 4

Ingredients:
- 1 pound boneless, skinless chicken breasts, thinly sliced
- 2 cups broccoli florets
- 1 bell pepper, thinly sliced
- 1 carrot, julienned
- 1 cup snap peas
- 3 tablespoons soy sauce
- 2 tablespoons hoisin sauce
- 1 tablespoon sesame oil
- 1 tablespoon cornstarch
- 2 tablespoons vegetable oil
- 2 cloves garlic, minced
- 1 teaspoon ginger, grated
- Cooked brown rice for serving

Directions:
1. In a bowl, mix soy sauce, hoisin sauce, sesame oil, and cornstarch to create the sauce.
2. Heat vegetable oil in a wok or large skillet over high heat.
3. Add sliced chicken and stir-fry until browned and cooked through. Remove from the wok and set aside.
4. In the same wok, add a bit more oil if needed. Sauté garlic and ginger until fragrant.
5. Add broccoli, bell pepper, carrot, and snap peas to the wok. Stir-fry until vegetables are crisp-tender.
6. Return cooked chicken to the wok and pour the sauce over the chicken and vegetables. Toss to coat evenly.
7. Serve the Chicken and Vegetable Stir-Fry over cooked brown rice.

Nutritional Information (per serving):
- Calories: 320
- Protein: 25g

- Carbohydrates: 20g
- Fat: 15g
- Fiber: 4g

Quinoa and Roasted Vegetable Bowl

Nourish your body with the Quinoa and Roasted Vegetable Bowl, a wholesome combination of protein-packed quinoa and a medley of colorful roasted vegetables. This bowl is not only nutritious but also bursting with flavors and textures.

Total Time: 30 minutes
Servings: 4

Ingredients:
- 1 cup quinoa, cooked
- 1 sweet potato, peeled and diced
- 1 zucchini, sliced
- 1 red onion, thinly sliced
- 1 bell pepper, diced
- 2 tablespoons olive oil
- 1 teaspoon cumin
- 1 teaspoon smoked paprika
- Salt and pepper to taste
- 1 cup cherry tomatoes, halved
- 1/4 cup feta cheese, crumbled
- Fresh parsley for garnish

Directions:
1. Preheat the oven to 400°F (200°C).
2. In a bowl, toss diced sweet potato, sliced zucchini, thinly sliced red onion, and diced bell pepper with olive oil, cumin, smoked paprika, salt, and pepper.
3. Spread the vegetables on a baking sheet in a single layer.
4. Roast in the oven for 20-25 minutes or until the vegetables are tender and slightly caramelized.
5. In serving bowls, assemble the Quinoa and Roasted Vegetable Bowl by layering cooked quinoa and the roasted vegetables.
6. Top with halved cherry tomatoes, crumbled feta cheese, and fresh parsley.
7. Serve the bowl warm and enjoy the delightful combination of flavors.

Nutritional Information (per serving):
- Calories: 320
- Protein: 10g
- Carbohydrates: 50g
- Fat: 10g
- Fiber: 8g

Greek Salad with Grilled Salmon

Indulge in the flavors of the Mediterranean with the Greek Salad featuring Grilled Salmon. This vibrant salad combines crisp vegetables, tangy feta, Kalamata olives, and perfectly grilled salmon for a satisfying and healthy lunch.

Total Time: 30 minutes
Servings: 2

Ingredients:
- 2 salmon fillets
- 6 cups mixed salad greens
- 1 cucumber, sliced
- 1 cup cherry tomatoes, halved
- 1/2 red onion, thinly sliced
- 1/2 cup Kalamata olives, sliced
- 1/2 cup feta cheese, crumbled
- 2 tablespoons extra-virgin olive oil
- 1 tablespoon red wine vinegar
- 1 teaspoon dried oregano
- Salt and pepper to taste
- Lemon wedges for serving

Directions:
1. Preheat the grill or grill pan over medium-high heat.
2. Season salmon fillets with salt and pepper.
3. Grill salmon for 4-5 minutes per side or until cooked through.
4. In a large bowl, combine mixed salad greens, sliced cucumber, halved cherry tomatoes, thinly sliced red onion, Kalamata olives, and crumbled feta.
5. In a small bowl, whisk together olive oil, red wine vinegar, dried oregano, salt, and pepper.
6. Drizzle the dressing over the salad and toss gently to combine.
7. Divide the salad among plates and top each with a grilled salmon fillet.

8. Serve the Greek Salad with Grilled Salmon, accompanied by lemon wedges for a burst of citrus flavor.

Nutritional Information (per serving):
- Calories: 400
- Protein: 30g
- Carbohydrates: 20g
- Fat: 25g
- Fiber: 6g

Dinner

Baked Cod with Lemon and Herbs

Elevate your dinner with the light and flavorful Baked Cod with Lemon and Herbs. This dish features succulent cod fillets seasoned with zesty lemon and aromatic herbs, creating a delightful and nutritious main course.

Total Time: 25 minutes
Servings: 4

Ingredients:
- 4 cod fillets
- 2 tablespoons olive oil
- 2 tablespoons fresh lemon juice
- 2 cloves garlic, minced
- 1 teaspoon dried oregano
- 1 teaspoon dried thyme
- Salt and pepper to taste
- Lemon wedges for serving
- Fresh parsley for garnish

Directions:
1. Preheat the oven to 400°F (200°C).
2. Place cod fillets on a baking sheet lined with parchment paper.
3. In a bowl, whisk together olive oil, lemon juice, minced garlic, dried oregano, dried thyme, salt, and pepper.
4. Brush the cod fillets with the lemon and herb mixture, ensuring they are evenly coated.
5. Bake in the preheated oven for 15-18 minutes or until the cod is flaky and cooked through.
6. Serve the Baked Cod with Lemon and Herbs hot, garnished with lemon wedges and fresh parsley.

Nutritional Information (per serving):
- Calories: 200
- Protein: 25g
- Carbohydrates: 1g
- Fat: 10g
- Fiber: 0g

Cauliflower Rice Stir-Fry with Tofu

Experience a delicious and healthy dinner with the Cauliflower Rice Stir-Fry featuring tofu and an array of colorful vegetables. This low-carb alternative to traditional rice stir-fry is packed with protein and flavor.

Total Time: 30 minutes
Servings: 4

Ingredients:
- 1 block extra-firm tofu, pressed and cubed
- 1 medium cauliflower, grated into rice-like texture
- 1 bell pepper, thinly sliced
- 1 carrot, julienned
- 1 cup snap peas
- 3 tablespoons soy sauce
- 1 tablespoon sesame oil
- 1 tablespoon rice vinegar
- 1 teaspoon ginger, grated
- 2 cloves garlic, minced
- 2 green onions, sliced
- Sesame seeds for garnish

Directions:
1. In a wok or large skillet, sauté cubed tofu until golden brown. Set aside.
2. In the same wok, add a bit of oil and stir-fry bell pepper, julienned carrot, and snap peas until crisp-tender.
3. Add grated cauliflower to the vegetables and stir-fry for an additional 3-5 minutes.
4. In a small bowl, whisk together soy sauce, sesame oil, rice vinegar, grated ginger, and minced garlic.
5. Pour the sauce over the cauliflower and vegetable mixture. Add the cooked tofu and toss to combine.
6. Garnish with sliced green onions and sesame seeds before serving this Cauliflower Rice Stir-Fry with Tofu.

Nutritional Information (per serving):
- Calories: 220
- Protein: 15g
- Carbohydrates: 15g
- Fat: 12g
- Fiber: 7g

Spaghetti Squash with Turkey Bolognese

Enjoy a satisfying and nutritious dinner with Spaghetti Squash with Turkey Bolognese. This low-carb alternative to traditional pasta is paired with a flavorful turkey Bolognese sauce, creating a hearty and wholesome meal.

Total Time: 50 minutes
Servings: 4

Ingredients:

- 1 large spaghetti squash, halved and seeds removed
- 1 pound ground turkey
- 1 onion, diced
- 2 carrots, peeled and diced
- 2 celery stalks, diced
- 3 cloves garlic, minced
- 1 can (14 oz) crushed tomatoes
- 1/4 cup tomato paste
- 1 teaspoon dried oregano
- 1 teaspoon dried basil
- Salt and pepper to taste
- Fresh basil for garnish
- Parmesan cheese for serving

Directions:

1. Preheat the oven to 375°F (190°C).
2. Place spaghetti squash halves on a baking sheet, cut side down. Roast for 35-40 minutes or until the squash is fork-tender.
3. While the squash is roasting, in a large skillet, brown ground turkey over medium heat.
4. Add diced onion, carrots, celery, and minced garlic to the skillet. Sauté until vegetables are softened.
5. Stir in crushed tomatoes, tomato paste, dried oregano, dried basil, salt, and pepper. Simmer for 15-20 minutes.
6. Use a fork to scrape the cooked spaghetti squash into "noodles."
7. Serve the Spaghetti Squash with Turkey Bolognese over the squash noodles, garnished with fresh basil and Parmesan cheese.

Nutritional Information (per serving):

- Calories: 300
- Protein: 20g

- Carbohydrates: 30g
- Fat: 12g
- Fiber: 7g

Grilled Portobello Mushrooms with Quinoa

Delight your palate with the earthy flavors of Grilled Portobello Mushrooms paired with a bed of fluffy quinoa. This vegetarian dinner option is not only delicious but also a source of protein and essential nutrients.

Total Time: 35 minutes
Servings: 4

Ingredients:
- 4 large Portobello mushrooms, stems removed
- 1 cup quinoa, cooked
- 1 red bell pepper, sliced
- 1 zucchini, sliced
- 2 tablespoons balsamic vinegar
- 2 tablespoons olive oil
- 2 cloves garlic, minced
- 1 teaspoon dried thyme
- Salt and pepper to taste
- Fresh parsley for garnish

Directions:
1. Preheat the grill or grill pan over medium-high heat.
2. In a bowl, whisk together balsamic vinegar, olive oil, minced garlic, dried thyme, salt, and pepper.
3. Brush the Portobello mushrooms, red bell pepper, and zucchini with the balsamic mixture.
4. Grill the mushrooms for 4-5 minutes per side, until tender.
5. Grill the red bell pepper and zucchini until charred and crisp-tender.
6. In serving plates, assemble Grilled Portobello Mushrooms over a bed of cooked quinoa, surrounded by grilled vegetables.
7. Garnish with fresh parsley and serve this delightful vegetarian dish.

Nutritional Information (per serving):
- Calories: 250
- Protein: 8g

- Carbohydrates: 35g
- Fat: 10g
- Fiber: 6g

Lemon Herb Chicken Skewers

Transform your dinner into a culinary delight with Lemon Herb Chicken Skewers. These skewers are marinated in a zesty lemon and herb mixture, creating a flavorful and protein-packed dish that is perfect for grilling or baking.

Total Time: 30 minutes (plus marinating time)
Servings: 4

Ingredients:
- 1.5 pounds boneless, skinless chicken breasts, cut into cubes
- 1/4 cup olive oil
- 3 tablespoons fresh lemon juice
- 2 cloves garlic, minced
- 1 teaspoon dried oregano
- 1 teaspoon dried thyme
- 1 teaspoon dried rosemary
- Salt and pepper to taste
- Lemon wedges for serving
- Fresh parsley for garnish

Directions:
1. In a bowl, whisk together olive oil, fresh lemon juice, minced garlic, dried oregano, dried thyme, dried rosemary, salt, and pepper.
2. Place chicken cubes in a resealable plastic bag and pour the marinade over them. Seal the bag and refrigerate for at least 2 hours, or overnight for best flavor.
3. Preheat the grill or grill pan over medium-high heat.
4. Thread marinated chicken cubes onto skewers.
5. Grill the chicken skewers for 6-8 minutes per side, or until fully cooked.
6. Serve the Lemon Herb Chicken Skewers hot, garnished with lemon wedges and fresh parsley.

Nutritional Information (per serving):
- Calories: 280
- Protein: 30g
- Carbohydrates: 2g

- Fat: 16g
- Fiber: 1g

Eggplant Lasagna with Ground Turkey

Indulge in a lighter twist on traditional lasagna with the Eggplant Lasagna featuring savory ground turkey. Layers of thinly sliced eggplant replace traditional noodles, creating a wholesome and delicious dinner option.

Total Time: 1 hour
Servings: 6

Ingredients:
- 1 large eggplant, thinly sliced lengthwise
- 1 pound ground turkey
- 1 onion, diced
- 2 cloves garlic, minced
- 1 can (14 oz) crushed tomatoes
- 1 can (6 oz) tomato paste
- 1 teaspoon dried oregano
- 1 teaspoon dried basil
- Salt and pepper to taste
- 2 cups ricotta cheese
- 2 cups shredded mozzarella cheese
- 1/2 cup grated Parmesan cheese
- Fresh basil for garnish

Directions:
1. Preheat the oven to 375°F (190°C).
2. In a skillet, brown ground turkey over medium heat. Add diced onion and minced garlic, sautéing until the onion is translucent.
3. Stir in crushed tomatoes, tomato paste, dried oregano, dried basil, salt, and pepper. Simmer for 15 minutes.
4. In a separate bowl, combine ricotta cheese, shredded mozzarella cheese, and grated Parmesan cheese.
5. In a baking dish, layer sliced eggplant, followed by the turkey and tomato sauce, and the cheese mixture. Repeat until the dish is filled, finishing with a layer of cheese on top.
6. Bake in the preheated oven for 40-45 minutes or until the eggplant is tender and the cheese is bubbly and golden.

7. Garnish with fresh basil before serving this Eggplant Lasagna with Ground Turkey.

Nutritional Information (per serving):
- Calories: 350
- Protein: 25g
- Carbohydrates: 15g
- Fat: 20g
- Fiber: 5g

Salmon with Dill and Lemon

Elevate your dinner with the simplicity of Salmon with Dill and Lemon. This dish highlights the natural flavors of salmon, enhanced with the brightness of dill and lemon, creating a quick and nutritious meal.

Total Time: 20 minutes
Servings: 4

Ingredients:
- 4 salmon fillets
- 2 tablespoons fresh dill, chopped
- 1 lemon, thinly sliced
- 2 tablespoons olive oil
- Salt and pepper to taste
- Lemon wedges for serving

Directions:
1. Preheat the oven to 400°F (200°C).
2. Place salmon fillets on a baking sheet lined with parchment paper.
3. Drizzle olive oil over the salmon, ensuring each fillet is coated.
4. Sprinkle chopped dill over the salmon and season with salt and pepper.
5. Place lemon slices on top of each fillet.
6. Bake in the preheated oven for 15-18 minutes or until the salmon is cooked through and flakes easily with a fork.
7. Serve the Salmon with Dill and Lemon hot, accompanied by lemon wedges.

Nutritional Information (per serving):
- Calories: 300
- Protein: 30g

- Carbohydrates: 2g
- Fat: 20g
- Fiber: 1g

Turkey and Vegetable Meatballs

Enjoy a healthier take on classic meatballs with these Turkey and Vegetable Meatballs. Packed with lean ground turkey and colorful vegetables, these meatballs are a delicious and nutritious addition to your dinner.

Total Time: 40 minutes
Servings: 5 (4 meatballs per serving)

Ingredients:
- 1 pound ground turkey
- 1 zucchini, grated and excess water squeezed out
- 1 carrot, grated
- 1/2 onion, finely chopped
- 2 cloves garlic, minced
- 1/4 cup breadcrumbs (whole wheat or gluten-free)
- 1/4 cup grated Parmesan cheese
- 1 egg
- 2 tablespoons fresh parsley, chopped
- 1 teaspoon dried oregano
- Salt and pepper to taste
- Olive oil for cooking
- Marinara sauce for serving

Directions:
1. Preheat the oven to 375°F (190°C).
2. In a bowl, combine ground turkey, grated zucchini, grated carrot, chopped onion, minced garlic, breadcrumbs, Parmesan cheese, egg, fresh parsley, dried oregano, salt, and pepper.
3. Mix until all ingredients are well combined.
4. Form the mixture into meatballs and place them on a baking sheet lined with parchment paper.
5. Drizzle olive oil over the meatballs and bake in the preheated oven for 20-25 minutes or until they are cooked through and browned on the outside.
6. Serve the Turkey and Vegetable Meatballs with marinara sauce.

Nutritional Information (per serving):
- Calories: 250
- Protein: 20g
- Carbohydrates: 10g
- Fat: 15g
- Fiber: 2g

Stuffed Acorn Squash with Quinoa and Cranberries

Embrace the flavors of fall with Stuffed Acorn Squash featuring a hearty filling of quinoa, cranberries, and aromatic spices. This dish not only looks impressive but also offers a wholesome and satisfying dinner option.

Total Time: 1 hour
Servings: 4

Ingredients:
- 2 acorn squash, halved and seeds removed
- 1 cup quinoa, cooked
- 1/2 cup dried cranberries
- 1/4 cup chopped pecans
- 2 tablespoons maple syrup
- 1 teaspoon ground cinnamon
- 1/2 teaspoon ground nutmeg
- Salt and pepper to taste
- Olive oil for brushing
- Fresh parsley for garnish

Directions:
1. Preheat the oven to 375°F (190°C).
2. Brush the cut sides of the acorn squash with olive oil and place them on a baking sheet, cut side down.
3. Bake in the preheated oven for 30-40 minutes or until the squash is fork-tender.
4. In a bowl, combine cooked quinoa, dried cranberries, chopped pecans, maple syrup, ground cinnamon, ground nutmeg, salt, and pepper.
5. Flip the baked acorn squash halves and fill each cavity with the quinoa mixture.
6. Return the stuffed acorn squash to the oven and bake for an additional 15-20 minutes, allowing the flavors to meld.
7. Garnish with fresh parsley before serving this delightful Stuffed Acorn Squash with Quinoa and Cranberries.

Nutritional Information (per serving):
- Calories: 320
- Protein: 8g
- Carbohydrates: 60g
- Fat: 6g
- Fiber: 8g

Veggie-loaded Chicken Curry

Experience a burst of flavors with Veggie-loaded Chicken Curry, a wholesome and comforting dinner option. This curry is packed with colorful vegetables, tender chicken, and a fragrant blend of spices, creating a nutritious and satisfying meal.

Total Time: 45 minutes
Servings: 6

Ingredients:
- 1.5 pounds boneless, skinless chicken thighs, cut into cubes
- 1 onion, finely chopped
- 2 bell peppers, diced
- 1 zucchini, sliced
- 1 cup cauliflower florets
- 2 carrots, sliced
- 3 cloves garlic, minced
- 1 tablespoon ginger, grated
- 2 tablespoons curry powder
- 1 teaspoon ground turmeric
- 1 teaspoon ground cumin
- 1 can (14 oz) coconut milk
- 1 can (14 oz) diced tomatoes
- Salt and pepper to taste
- Fresh cilantro for garnish
- Cooked brown rice for serving

Directions:
1. In a large pot or Dutch oven, sauté chopped onion, minced garlic, and grated ginger until fragrant.
2. Add cubed chicken to the pot and brown on all sides.
3. Stir in curry powder, ground turmeric, and ground cumin, coating the chicken with the spices.

4. Add diced bell peppers, sliced zucchini, cauliflower florets, sliced carrots, coconut milk, and diced tomatoes to the pot. Season with salt and pepper.
5. Bring the curry to a boil, then reduce heat and simmer for 25-30 minutes or until the vegetables are tender and the chicken is cooked through.
6. Serve the Veggie-loaded Chicken Curry over cooked brown rice, garnished with fresh cilantro.

Nutritional Information (per serving):
- Calories: 350
- Protein: 25g
- Carbohydrates: 20g
- Fat: 18g
- Fiber: 6g

Quinoa-stuffed Bell Peppers

Elevate your dinner with Quinoa-stuffed Bell Peppers, a colorful and nutritious dish that combines the wholesome goodness of quinoa with the vibrant flavors of bell peppers. This meal is a delightful way to enjoy a variety of vegetables and protein in one flavorful package.

Total Time: 45 minutes
Servings: 4

Ingredients:
- 4 bell peppers, halved and seeds removed
- 1 cup quinoa, cooked
- 1 can (15 oz) black beans, drained and rinsed
- 1 cup corn kernels
- 1 cup cherry tomatoes, halved
- 1/2 cup red onion, finely chopped
- 1 cup shredded cheddar cheese
- 2 tablespoons olive oil
- 1 teaspoon cumin
- 1 teaspoon chili powder
- Salt and pepper to taste
- Fresh cilantro for garnish

Directions:
1. Preheat the oven to 375°F (190°C).
2. In a bowl, combine cooked quinoa, black beans, corn kernels, cherry tomatoes, red onion, shredded cheddar cheese, olive oil, cumin, chili powder, salt, and pepper.
3. Stuff each bell pepper half with the quinoa mixture, pressing down gently.
4. Place the stuffed bell peppers in a baking dish and cover with aluminum foil.
5. Bake in the preheated oven for 25-30 minutes or until the peppers are tender.
6. Remove the foil and bake for an additional 5-10 minutes to melt the cheese and lightly brown the tops.
7. Garnish with fresh cilantro before serving these delightful Quinoa-stuffed Bell Peppers.

Nutritional Information (per serving):
- Calories: 350
- Protein: 15g
- Carbohydrates: 50g
- Fat: 12g
- Fiber: 10g

Shrimp and Broccoli Stir-Fry

Experience the perfect balance of flavors and textures with Shrimp and Broccoli Stir-Fry. This quick and easy dinner option combines succulent shrimp, crisp broccoli, and a savory stir-fry sauce, creating a delicious and nutritious meal in no time.

Total Time: 20 minutes
Servings: 3

Ingredients:
- 1 pound shrimp, peeled and deveined
- 4 cups broccoli florets
- 1 red bell pepper, sliced
- 2 tablespoons soy sauce
- 1 tablespoon oyster sauce
- 1 tablespoon hoisin sauce
- 1 tablespoon sesame oil
- 2 tablespoons vegetable oil
- 3 cloves garlic, minced
- 1 teaspoon ginger, grated

- Cooked brown rice for serving
- Sesame seeds for garnish

Directions:
1. In a bowl, mix together soy sauce, oyster sauce, hoisin sauce, and sesame oil to create the stir-fry sauce.
2. Heat vegetable oil in a wok or large skillet over high heat.
3. Add minced garlic and grated ginger, stir-frying until fragrant.
4. Add shrimp to the wok and cook until pink and opaque. Remove shrimp from the wok and set aside.
5. In the same wok, stir-fry broccoli and sliced red bell pepper until crisp-tender.
6. Return the cooked shrimp to the wok and pour the stir-fry sauce over the mixture. Toss to coat evenly.
7. Serve the Shrimp and Broccoli Stir-Fry over cooked brown rice, garnished with sesame seeds.

Nutritional Information (per serving):
- Calories: 300
- Protein: 25g
- Carbohydrates: 20g
- Fat: 12g
- Fiber: 5g

Baked Sweet Potato with Chickpea Salad

Enjoy a nutritious and satisfying dinner with Baked Sweet Potato topped with a flavorful Chickpea Salad. This dish combines the natural sweetness of sweet potatoes with the protein-rich goodness of chickpeas and a medley of fresh ingredients.

Total Time: 50 minutes
Servings: 4

Ingredients:
- 4 large sweet potatoes
- 2 cans (15 oz each) chickpeas, drained and rinsed
- 1 cucumber, diced
- 1 bell pepper, diced
- 1/2 red onion, finely chopped
- 1/4 cup fresh parsley, chopped
- 1/4 cup feta cheese, crumbled

- 2 tablespoons olive oil
- 1 tablespoon red wine vinegar
- Salt and pepper to taste
- Greek yogurt for serving

Directions:
1. Preheat the oven to 400°F (200°C).
2. Wash and prick sweet potatoes with a fork. Place them on a baking sheet and bake for 40-45 minutes or until tender.
3. In a bowl, combine chickpeas, diced cucumber, diced bell pepper, chopped red onion, fresh parsley, crumbled feta cheese, olive oil, red wine vinegar, salt, and pepper.
4. Cut a slit in each baked sweet potato and fluff the flesh with a fork.
5. Top each sweet potato with the chickpea salad.
6. Serve the Baked Sweet Potato with Chickpea Salad, accompanied by a dollop of Greek yogurt if desired.

Nutritional Information (per serving):
- Calories: 350
- Protein: 12g
- Carbohydrates: 60g
- Fat: 8g
- Fiber: 12g

Roasted Brussels Sprouts and Salmon

Delight your taste buds with the exquisite pairing of Roasted Brussels Sprouts and Salmon. This dinner option not only offers a burst of flavors but also provides a healthy dose of omega-3 fatty acids and essential nutrients.

Total Time: 30 minutes
Servings: 2

Ingredients:
- 2 salmon fillets
- 2 cups Brussels sprouts, halved
- 2 tablespoons olive oil
- 1 tablespoon balsamic vinegar
- 1 teaspoon Dijon mustard
- 2 cloves garlic, minced

- Salt and pepper to taste
- Lemon wedges for serving

Directions:
1. Preheat the oven to 400°F (200°C).
2. In a bowl, whisk together olive oil, balsamic vinegar, Dijon mustard, minced garlic, salt, and pepper.
3. Place Brussels sprouts on a baking sheet and toss with half of the prepared dressing.
4. Push the Brussels sprouts to the edges of the baking sheet, creating space for the salmon fillets in the center.
5. Place the salmon fillets on the baking sheet and drizzle them with the remaining dressing.
6. Roast in the preheated oven for 15-20 minutes or until the salmon is cooked through and the Brussels sprouts are crispy.
7. Serve the Roasted Brussels Sprouts and Salmon hot, accompanied by lemon wedges for a touch of citrus.

Nutritional Information (per serving):
- Calories: 400
- Protein: 30g
- Carbohydrates: 20g
- Fat: 22g
- Fiber: 8g

Turkey and Vegetable Kabobs

Experience the joy of grilling with Turkey and Vegetable Kabobs, a dinner option that combines lean turkey with a colorful array of vegetables. These kabobs are not only visually appealing but also a tasty and healthy choice for a delightful evening meal.

Total Time: 35 minutes
Servings: 4

Ingredients:
- 1.5 pounds ground turkey
- 1 bell pepper, cut into chunks
- 1 zucchini, sliced
- 1 red onion, cut into chunks
- 1 cup cherry tomatoes

- 2 tablespoons olive oil
- 1 tablespoon fresh lemon juice
- 1 teaspoon dried oregano
- 1 teaspoon smoked paprika
- Salt and pepper to taste
- Wooden or metal skewers

Directions:

1. Preheat the grill or grill pan over medium-high heat.
2. In a bowl, combine ground turkey, olive oil, fresh lemon juice, dried oregano, smoked paprika, salt, and pepper. Mix until well combined.
3. Form the turkey mixture into small meatballs.
4. Thread the turkey meatballs, bell pepper chunks, zucchini slices, red onion chunks, and cherry tomatoes onto skewers, alternating the ingredients.
5. Grill the kabobs for 12-15 minutes, turning occasionally, until the turkey is cooked through and the vegetables are tender.
6. Serve the Turkey and Vegetable Kabobs hot, with your favorite dipping sauce if desired.

Nutritional Information (per serving):

- Calories: 320
- Protein: 25g
- Carbohydrates: 15g
- Fat: 18g
- Fiber: 5g

Vegetables

Garlic Roasted Asparagus

Elevate the natural flavor of asparagus with the simplicity of Garlic Roasted Asparagus. This side dish is not only easy to prepare but also brings out the vibrant taste of asparagus with the aromatic touch of roasted garlic.

Total Time: 20 minutes
Servings: 4

Ingredients:
- 1 pound asparagus, trimmed
- 2 tablespoons olive oil
- 3 cloves garlic, minced
- Salt and pepper to taste
- Lemon wedges for serving (optional)

Directions:
1. Preheat the oven to 425°F (220°C).
2. Place trimmed asparagus on a baking sheet.
3. Drizzle olive oil over the asparagus, ensuring they are evenly coated.
4. Sprinkle minced garlic, salt, and pepper over the asparagus, tossing to combine.
5. Roast in the preheated oven for 12-15 minutes or until the asparagus is tender but still crisp.
6. Serve the Garlic Roasted Asparagus hot, with optional lemon wedges on the side.

Nutritional Information (per serving):
- Calories: 80
- Protein: 3g
- Carbohydrates: 6g
- Fat: 6g
- Fiber: 3g

Lemon Herb Roasted Zucchini

Bring a burst of freshness to your plate with Lemon Herb Roasted Zucchini. This side dish combines the delicate flavors of zucchini with zesty lemon and aromatic herbs, creating a light and flavorful addition to any meal.

Total Time: 25 minutes
Servings: 4

Ingredients:
- 4 medium zucchini, sliced
- 2 tablespoons olive oil
- 2 tablespoons fresh lemon juice
- 1 teaspoon dried thyme
- 1 teaspoon dried rosemary
- Salt and pepper to taste
- Fresh parsley for garnish

Directions:
1. Preheat the oven to 400°F (200°C).
2. Place sliced zucchini on a baking sheet.
3. In a bowl, whisk together olive oil, fresh lemon juice, dried thyme, dried rosemary, salt, and pepper.
4. Drizzle the lemon herb mixture over the zucchini, tossing to coat evenly.
5. Roast in the preheated oven for 15-18 minutes or until the zucchini is golden and tender.
6. Garnish with fresh parsley before serving this delightful Lemon Herb Roasted Zucchini.

Nutritional Information (per serving):
- Calories: 90
- Protein: 2g
- Carbohydrates: 7g
- Fat: 7g
- Fiber: 2g

Sauteed Spinach with Garlic and Olive Oil

Enjoy the simplicity of Sauteed Spinach with Garlic and Olive Oil, a classic side dish that lets the natural goodness of spinach shine. This quick and easy recipe brings out the rich flavors of garlic and olive oil, complementing the tender spinach leaves.

Total Time: 10 minutes
Servings: 4

Ingredients:
- 1 pound fresh spinach, washed and trimmed
- 2 tablespoons olive oil
- 3 cloves garlic, minced
- Salt and pepper to taste
- Lemon wedges for serving (optional)

Directions:
1. In a large skillet, heat olive oil over medium heat.
2. Add minced garlic to the skillet, sautéing until fragrant.
3. Add fresh spinach to the skillet in batches, tossing until wilted.
4. Season with salt and pepper, continuing to sauté until the spinach is tender.
5. Serve the Sauteed Spinach hot, with optional lemon wedges on the side.

Nutritional Information (per serving):
- Calories: 70
- Protein: 4g
- Carbohydrates: 3g
- Fat: 5g
- Fiber: 2g

Balsamic Glazed Brussels Sprouts

Transform Brussels sprouts into a delectable side dish with Balsamic Glazed Brussels Sprouts. This recipe combines the nutty flavor of Brussels sprouts with a sweet and tangy balsamic glaze, creating a dish that is both savory and satisfying.

Total Time: 30 minutes
Servings: 4

Ingredients:
- 1 pound Brussels sprouts, trimmed and halved
- 2 tablespoons olive oil
- 2 tablespoons balsamic vinegar
- 1 tablespoon honey
- Salt and pepper to taste
- Toasted pine nuts for garnish (optional)

Directions:
1. Preheat the oven to 400°F (200°C).
2. Place halved Brussels sprouts on a baking sheet.
3. In a bowl, whisk together olive oil, balsamic vinegar, honey, salt, and pepper.
4. Drizzle the balsamic mixture over the Brussels sprouts, tossing to coat evenly.
5. Roast in the preheated oven for 20-25 minutes or until the Brussels sprouts are caramelized and golden.
6. Garnish with toasted pine nuts if desired before serving these delightful Balsamic Glazed Brussels Sprouts.

Nutritional Information (per serving):
- Calories: 120
- Protein: 4g
- Carbohydrates: 18g
- Fat: 5g
- Fiber: 5g

Roasted Root Vegetables with Rosemary

Experience the warmth and comfort of Roasted Root Vegetables with Rosemary. This side dish combines a medley of hearty root vegetables with the earthy aroma of rosemary, creating a wholesome and flavorful addition to your dinner table.

Total Time: 45 minutes
Servings: 6

Ingredients:
- 2 cups baby potatoes, halved
- 2 cups carrots, peeled and sliced
- 2 cups parsnips, peeled and sliced
- 2 tablespoons olive oil
- 1 tablespoon fresh rosemary, chopped

- Salt and pepper to taste
- Fresh parsley for garnish

Directions:
1. Preheat the oven to 425°F (220°C).
2. Place halved baby potatoes, sliced carrots, and sliced parsnips on a baking sheet.
3. Drizzle olive oil over the vegetables, tossing to coat evenly.
4. Sprinkle chopped fresh rosemary, salt, and pepper over the vegetables, mixing well.
5. Roast in the preheated oven for 30-35 minutes or until the vegetables are golden and tender.
6. Garnish with fresh parsley before serving these delightful Roasted Root Vegetables with Rosemary.

Nutritional Information (per serving):
- Calories: 150
- Protein: 2g
- Carbohydrates: 25g
- Fat: 6g
- Fiber: 5g

Cucumber and Tomato Salad with Dill

Refresh your palate with the vibrant flavors of Cucumber and Tomato Salad with Dill. This light and crisp salad brings together the freshness of cucumber and tomatoes, enhanced by the aromatic touch of dill, creating a perfect side dish for any meal.

Total Time: 15 minutes
Servings: 4

Ingredients:
- 2 cucumbers, thinly sliced
- 2 cups cherry tomatoes, halved
- 2 tablespoons fresh dill, chopped
- 3 tablespoons olive oil
- 1 tablespoon red wine vinegar
- Salt and pepper to taste
- Feta cheese for garnish (optional)

Directions:
1. In a large bowl, combine sliced cucumbers, halved cherry tomatoes, and chopped fresh dill.
2. In a small bowl, whisk together olive oil, red wine vinegar, salt, and pepper.
3. Drizzle the dressing over the cucumber and tomato mixture, tossing gently to coat.
4. Garnish with crumbled feta cheese if desired before serving this refreshing Cucumber and Tomato Salad with Dill.

Nutritional Information (per serving):
- Calories: 120
- Protein: 2g
- Carbohydrates: 8g
- Fat: 10g
- Fiber: 2g

Grilled Eggplant with Tahini Sauce

Elevate the humble eggplant with the rich and nutty flavors of Grilled Eggplant with Tahini Sauce. This dish combines smoky grilled eggplant with a creamy tahini sauce, creating a delightful side that is both satisfying and flavorful.

Total Time: 30 minutes
Servings: 4

Ingredients:
- 2 large eggplants, sliced
- 1/4 cup olive oil
- Salt and pepper to taste
- Sesame seeds for garnish
- Fresh parsley for garnish

Tahini Sauce:
- 1/2 cup tahini
- 2 tablespoons lemon juice
- 2 cloves garlic, minced
- 2 tablespoons water
- Salt to taste

Directions:
1. Preheat the grill or grill pan over medium-high heat.

2. Brush eggplant slices with olive oil and season with salt and pepper.
3. Grill the eggplant slices for 3-4 minutes per side or until tender and grill marks appear.
4. In a small bowl, whisk together tahini, lemon juice, minced garlic, water, and salt to create the tahini sauce.
5. Arrange grilled eggplant slices on a serving platter, drizzling tahini sauce over them.
6. Garnish with sesame seeds and fresh parsley before serving this flavorful Grilled Eggplant with Tahini Sauce.

Nutritional Information (per serving):
- Calories: 200
- Protein: 4g
- Carbohydrates: 12g
- Fat: 15g
- Fiber: 6g

Steamed Broccoli with Almond Slivers

Keep it simple yet nutritious with Steamed Broccoli with Almond Slivers. This side dish brings out the vibrant green color and natural crunch of broccoli, complemented by the nutty flavor of slivered almonds.

Total Time: 10 minutes
Servings: 4

Ingredients:
- 4 cups broccoli florets
- 1/4 cup almond slivers
- 2 tablespoons olive oil
- 1 tablespoon lemon juice
- Salt and pepper to taste
- Lemon zest for garnish

Directions:
1. Steam broccoli florets until tender-crisp, about 5 minutes.
2. In a dry skillet, toast almond slivers over medium heat until golden and fragrant.
3. In a bowl, toss steamed broccoli with toasted almond slivers, olive oil, lemon juice, salt, and pepper.

4. Garnish with lemon zest before serving this simple and nutritious Steamed Broccoli with Almond Slivers.

Nutritional Information (per serving):
- Calories: 120
- Protein: 4g
- Carbohydrates: 10g
- Fat: 8g
- Fiber: 4g

Stir-Fried Green Beans with Sesame Seeds

Enjoy the crispiness of green beans in a flavorful Stir-Fried Green Beans with Sesame Seeds. This side dish combines the freshness of green beans with the nutty aroma of sesame seeds, creating a quick and tasty addition to your meal.

Total Time: 15 minutes
Servings: 4

Ingredients:
- 1 pound green beans, trimmed
- 2 tablespoons sesame oil
- 2 tablespoons soy sauce
- 1 tablespoon rice vinegar
- 1 tablespoon honey
- 2 cloves garlic, minced
- 2 tablespoons sesame seeds, toasted
- Red pepper flakes for garnish (optional)

Directions:
1. In a wok or large skillet, heat sesame oil over medium-high heat.
2. Add trimmed green beans to the wok, stir-frying for 5-7 minutes or until they are tender-crisp.
3. In a small bowl, whisk together soy sauce, rice vinegar, honey, and minced garlic.
4. Pour the sauce over the green beans, tossing to coat evenly.
5. Sprinkle toasted sesame seeds over the stir-fried green beans.
6. Garnish with red pepper flakes if desired before serving this delicious Stir-Fried Green Beans with Sesame Seeds.

Nutritional Information (per serving):
- Calories: 90
- Protein: 2g
- Carbohydrates: 10g
- Fat: 5g
- Fiber: 3g

Mashed Cauliflower with Garlic

Experience the comfort of mashed potatoes with a healthier twist in Mashed Cauliflower with Garlic. This side dish replaces traditional mashed potatoes with cauliflower, creating a creamy and flavorful alternative that is both satisfying and nutritious.

Total Time: 20 minutes
Servings: 4

Ingredients:
- 1 large head cauliflower, cut into florets
- 3 cloves garlic, minced
- 2 tablespoons butter
- 1/4 cup milk (dairy or plant-based)
- Salt and pepper to taste
- Chopped chives for garnish

Directions:
1. Steam cauliflower florets until very tender, about 10 minutes.
2. In a food processor, combine steamed cauliflower, minced garlic, butter, and milk.
3. Blend until smooth and creamy. Add more milk if needed to reach the desired consistency.
4. Season with salt and pepper to taste.
5. Garnish with chopped chives before serving this delightful Mashed Cauliflower with Garlic.

Nutritional Information (per serving):
- Calories: 80
- Protein: 3g
- Carbohydrates: 10g
- Fat: 4g
- Fiber: 4g

Soups

Butternut Squash Soup with Apple

Embrace the flavors of fall with Butternut Squash Soup with Apple. This velvety soup combines the sweetness of butternut squash with the tartness of apple, creating a comforting and nourishing bowl perfect for chilly days.

Total Time: 45 minutes
Servings: 6

Ingredients:
- 1 medium butternut squash, peeled and diced
- 2 apples, peeled, cored, and diced
- 1 onion, chopped
- 2 carrots, chopped
- 4 cups vegetable broth
- 1 teaspoon curry powder
- 1/2 teaspoon cinnamon
- Salt and pepper to taste
- 1 cup coconut milk
- Fresh sage leaves for garnish

Directions:
1. In a large pot, sauté chopped onion in olive oil until translucent.
2. Add diced butternut squash, apples, carrots, vegetable broth, curry powder, cinnamon, salt, and pepper to the pot.
3. Bring to a boil, then reduce heat and simmer for 25-30 minutes or until vegetables are tender.
4. Use an immersion blender to puree the soup until smooth.
5. Stir in coconut milk and heat through.
6. Garnish with fresh sage leaves before serving this delightful Butternut Squash Soup with Apple.

Nutritional Information (per serving):
- Calories: 180
- Protein: 2g
- Carbohydrates: 30g
- Fat: 8g
- Fiber: 5g

Chicken and Rice Soup

Find comfort in a classic with Chicken and Rice Soup. This hearty and wholesome soup combines tender chicken, rice, and a medley of vegetables, creating a soothing bowl that's perfect for nourishing your body and soul.

Total Time: 40 minutes
Servings: 8

Ingredients:
- 1 pound boneless, skinless chicken breasts, diced
- 1 cup carrots, sliced
- 1 cup celery, diced
- 1 onion, chopped
- 2 cloves garlic, minced
- 8 cups chicken broth
- 1 cup white rice, uncooked
- 1 teaspoon dried thyme
- Salt and pepper to taste
- Fresh parsley for garnish

Directions:
1. In a large pot, sauté chopped onion and minced garlic until fragrant.
2. Add diced chicken, carrots, celery, chicken broth, rice, dried thyme, salt, and pepper to the pot.
3. Bring to a boil, then reduce heat and simmer for 20-25 minutes or until the chicken is cooked and rice is tender.
4. Adjust seasoning if needed and serve the Chicken and Rice Soup hot, garnished with fresh parsley.

Nutritional Information (per serving):
- Calories: 250
- Protein: 20g
- Carbohydrates: 30g
- Fat: 4g
- Fiber: 2g

Creamy Carrot and Ginger Soup

Indulge in the silky richness of Creamy Carrot and Ginger Soup. This vibrant and flavorful soup combines the sweetness of carrots with the warmth of ginger, creating a comforting and satisfying dish that's perfect for any occasion.

Total Time: 30 minutes
Servings: 6

Ingredients:
- 1 pound carrots, peeled and chopped
- 1 onion, chopped
- 2 tablespoons olive oil
- 1 tablespoon fresh ginger, grated
- 4 cups vegetable broth
- 1 cup coconut milk
- Salt and pepper to taste
- Fresh cilantro for garnish

Directions:
1. In a large pot, sauté chopped onion in olive oil until translucent.
2. Add chopped carrots, grated ginger, vegetable broth, salt, and pepper to the pot.
3. Bring to a boil, then reduce heat and simmer for 15-20 minutes or until carrots are tender.
4. Use an immersion blender to puree the soup until smooth.
5. Stir in coconut milk and heat through.
6. Garnish with fresh cilantro before serving this luscious Creamy Carrot and Ginger Soup.

Nutritional Information (per serving):
- Calories: 180
- Protein: 2g
- Carbohydrates: 15g
- Fat: 12g
- Fiber: 4g

Lentil and Kale Soup

Nourish your body with the wholesome goodness of Lentil and Kale Soup. Packed with protein-rich lentils and nutrient-dense kale, this soup is not only delicious but also a powerhouse of nutrition, making it an excellent choice for a satisfying meal.

Total Time: 45 minutes
Servings: 6

Ingredients:
- 1 cup green lentils, rinsed
- 1 onion, chopped
- 2 carrots, chopped
- 2 celery stalks, chopped
- 3 cloves garlic, minced
- 8 cups vegetable broth
- 1 can (14 oz) diced tomatoes
- 2 cups kale, chopped
- 1 teaspoon cumin
- 1 teaspoon paprika
- Salt and pepper to taste
- Lemon wedges for serving

Directions:
1. In a large pot, sauté chopped onion and minced garlic until fragrant.
2. Add green lentils, chopped carrots, chopped celery, vegetable broth, diced tomatoes, cumin, paprika, salt, and pepper to the pot.
3. Bring to a boil, then reduce heat and simmer for 30-35 minutes or until lentils are tender.
4. Stir in chopped kale and cook until wilted.
5. Adjust seasoning if needed and serve the Lentil and Kale Soup hot, with lemon wedges on the side.

Nutritional Information (per serving):
- Calories: 250
- Protein: 15g
- Carbohydrates: 40g
- Fat: 2g
- Fiber: 12g

Quinoa Minestrone Soup

Experience the hearty goodness of Quinoa Minestrone Soup. This wholesome soup combines the richness of tomatoes, the heartiness of quinoa, and a medley of vegetables, creating a satisfying and nutritious bowl that's perfect for a comforting meal.

Total Time: 35 minutes
Servings: 8

Ingredients:
- 1 cup quinoa, rinsed
- 1 onion, chopped
- 2 carrots, chopped
- 2 celery stalks, chopped
- 3 cloves garlic, minced
- 1 can (14 oz) diced tomatoes
- 8 cups vegetable broth
- 1 zucchini, diced
- 1 cup green beans, chopped
- 1 can (15 oz) kidney beans, drained and rinsed
- 1 teaspoon dried oregano
- 1 teaspoon dried basil
- Salt and pepper to taste
- Fresh basil for garnish

Directions:
1. In a large pot, sauté chopped onion and minced garlic until fragrant.
2. Add rinsed quinoa, chopped carrots, chopped celery, diced tomatoes, vegetable broth, diced zucchini, chopped green beans, kidney beans, dried oregano, dried basil, salt, and pepper to the pot.
3. Bring to a boil, then reduce heat and simmer for 20-25 minutes or until quinoa and vegetables are tender.
4. Adjust seasoning if needed and serve the Quinoa Minestrone Soup hot, garnished with fresh basil.

Nutritional Information (per serving):
- Calories: 280
- Protein: 10g
- Carbohydrates: 50g
- Fat: 4g
- Fiber: 8g

Turkey and Vegetable Noodle Soup

Savor the comforting warmth of Turkey and Vegetable Noodle Soup. This wholesome soup combines lean turkey, an assortment of vegetables, and hearty noodles, creating a nourishing bowl that's perfect for a cozy and satisfying meal.

Total Time: 45 minutes
Servings: 6

Ingredients:
- 1 pound ground turkey
- 1 onion, chopped
- 2 carrots, sliced
- 2 celery stalks, chopped
- 3 cloves garlic, minced
- 8 cups chicken broth
- 1 cup egg noodles, uncooked
- 1 teaspoon dried thyme
- Salt and pepper to taste
- Fresh parsley for garnish

Directions:
1. In a large pot, brown ground turkey over medium heat until cooked through.
2. Add chopped onion, sliced carrots, chopped celery, minced garlic, chicken broth, egg noodles, dried thyme, salt, and pepper to the pot.
3. Bring to a boil, then reduce heat and simmer for 20-25 minutes or until vegetables are tender and noodles are cooked.
4. Adjust seasoning if needed and serve the Turkey and Vegetable Noodle Soup hot, garnished with fresh parsley.

Nutritional Information (per serving):
- Calories: 300
- Protein: 20g
- Carbohydrates: 25g
- Fat: 12g
- Fiber: 4g

Sweet Potato and Coconut Soup

Indulge in the velvety richness of Sweet Potato and Coconut Soup. This delightful soup combines the natural sweetness of sweet potatoes with the creamy texture of coconut milk, creating a luxurious and satisfying bowl that's both comforting and flavorful.

Total Time: 40 minutes
Servings: 4

Ingredients:
- 2 large sweet potatoes, peeled and diced
- 1 onion, chopped
- 2 tablespoons olive oil
- 4 cups vegetable broth
- 1 can (14 oz) coconut milk
- 1 teaspoon curry powder
- 1/2 teaspoon ground cinnamon
- Salt and pepper to taste
- Fresh cilantro for garnish

Directions:
1. In a large pot, sauté chopped onion in olive oil until translucent.
2. Add diced sweet potatoes, vegetable broth, coconut milk, curry powder, ground cinnamon, salt, and pepper to the pot.
3. Bring to a boil, then reduce heat and simmer for 20-25 minutes or until sweet potatoes are tender.
4. Use an immersion blender to puree the soup until smooth.
5. Adjust seasoning if needed and serve the Sweet Potato and Coconut Soup hot, garnished with fresh cilantro.

Nutritional Information (per serving):
- Calories: 280
- Protein: 4g
- Carbohydrates: 30g
- Fat: 18g
- Fiber: 5g

Tomato Basil Soup with Quinoa

Enjoy a twist on a classic with Tomato Basil Soup with Quinoa. This hearty soup combines the richness of tomatoes and basil with the wholesome goodness of quinoa, creating a flavorful and nutritious bowl that's perfect for any season.

Total Time: 30 minutes
Servings: 4

Ingredients:
- 1 can (28 oz) crushed tomatoes
- 1 onion, chopped
- 2 cloves garlic, minced
- 4 cups vegetable broth
- 1/2 cup quinoa, rinsed
- 1 teaspoon dried basil
- Salt and pepper to taste
- Fresh basil leaves for garnish

Directions:
1. In a large pot, sauté chopped onion and minced garlic until fragrant.
2. Add crushed tomatoes, vegetable broth, rinsed quinoa, dried basil, salt, and pepper to the pot.
3. Bring to a boil, then reduce heat and simmer for 15-20 minutes or until quinoa is cooked.
4. Adjust seasoning if needed and serve the Tomato Basil Soup with Quinoa hot, garnished with fresh basil leaves.

Nutritional Information (per serving):
- Calories: 220
- Protein: 6g
- Carbohydrates: 40g
- Fat: 4g
- Fiber: 6g

Spinach and White Bean Soup

Nourish your body with the goodness of Spinach and White Bean Soup. This nutrient-packed soup combines the earthy flavor of white beans with the freshness of spinach, creating a wholesome and delicious bowl that's perfect for a light and satisfying meal.

Total Time: 35 minutes
Servings: 6

Ingredients:

- 2 cans (15 oz each) white beans, drained and rinsed
- 1 onion, chopped
- 2 carrots, sliced
- 2 celery stalks, chopped
- 3 cloves garlic, minced
- 6 cups vegetable broth
- 4 cups fresh spinach
- 1 teaspoon dried oregano
- 1/2 teaspoon red pepper flakes
- Salt and pepper to taste
- Grated Parmesan cheese for garnish (optional)

Directions:

1. In a large pot, sauté chopped onion and minced garlic until fragrant.
2. Add white beans, sliced carrots, chopped celery, vegetable broth, dried oregano, red pepper flakes, salt, and pepper to the pot.
3. Bring to a boil, then reduce heat and simmer for 20-25 minutes or until vegetables are tender.
4. Stir in fresh spinach and cook until wilted.
5. Adjust seasoning if needed and serve the Spinach and White Bean Soup hot, garnished with grated Parmesan cheese if desired.

Nutritional Information (per serving):

- Calories: 240
- Protein: 12g
- Carbohydrates: 40g
- Fat: 2g
- Fiber: 10g

Roasted Red Pepper and Lentil Soup

Delight your taste buds with the bold flavors of Roasted Red Pepper and Lentil Soup. This hearty soup combines the smokiness of roasted red peppers with the protein-packed goodness of lentils, creating a robust and satisfying bowl that's perfect for a nourishing meal.

Total Time: 45 minutes
Servings: 6

Ingredients:
- 2 cups red lentils, rinsed
- 3 roasted red peppers, peeled and chopped
- 1 onion, chopped
- 2 cloves garlic, minced
- 6 cups vegetable broth
- 1 teaspoon smoked paprika
- 1/2 teaspoon cayenne pepper
- Salt and pepper to taste
- Greek yogurt for garnish
- Fresh cilantro for garnish

Directions:
1. In a large pot, sauté chopped onion and minced garlic until fragrant.
2. Add rinsed red lentils, chopped roasted red peppers, vegetable broth, smoked paprika, cayenne pepper, salt, and pepper to the pot.
3. Bring to a boil, then reduce heat and simmer for 30-35 minutes or until lentils are tender.
4. Use an immersion blender to puree the soup until smooth.
5. Adjust seasoning if needed and serve the Roasted Red Pepper and Lentil Soup hot, garnished with a dollop of Greek yogurt and fresh cilantro.

Nutritional Information (per serving):
- Calories: 290
- Protein: 15g
- Carbohydrates: 45g
- Fat: 2g
- Fiber: 8g

Sides and Savory Snacks

Roasted Chickpeas with Rosemary

Elevate your snack game with Roasted Chickpeas with Rosemary. These crunchy and flavorful chickpeas are seasoned with aromatic rosemary, making them a delicious and satisfying savory snack that's perfect for any occasion.

Total Time: 40 minutes
Servings: 4

Ingredients:
- 2 cans (15 oz each) chickpeas, drained and rinsed
- 2 tablespoons olive oil
- 1 tablespoon fresh rosemary, chopped
- 1 teaspoon garlic powder
- 1/2 teaspoon cayenne pepper
- Salt and pepper to taste

Directions:
1. Preheat the oven to 400°F (200°C).
2. In a bowl, toss chickpeas with olive oil, chopped rosemary, garlic powder, cayenne pepper, salt, and pepper.
3. Spread chickpeas in a single layer on a baking sheet.
4. Roast in the preheated oven for 30-35 minutes or until chickpeas are golden and crispy.
5. Allow to cool slightly before serving these delightful Roasted Chickpeas with Rosemary.

Nutritional Information (per serving):
- Calories: 180
- Protein: 8g
- Carbohydrates: 28g
- Fat: 5g
- Fiber: 7g

Kale Chips with Parmesan

Experience the perfect blend of crunch and flavor with Kale Chips with Parmesan. These crispy kale chips are lightly seasoned with Parmesan cheese, creating a guilt-free and savory snack that's not only delicious but also packed with nutrients.

Total Time: 20 minutes
Servings: 4

Ingredients:
- 1 bunch kale, stems removed and leaves torn into pieces
- 2 tablespoons olive oil
- 1/4 cup Parmesan cheese, grated
- Salt and pepper to taste

Directions:
1. Preheat the oven to 350°F (175°C).
2. In a large bowl, toss kale leaves with olive oil, ensuring they are evenly coated.
3. Spread kale in a single layer on a baking sheet.
4. Sprinkle grated Parmesan cheese, salt, and pepper over the kale.
5. Bake in the preheated oven for 10-15 minutes or until kale is crisp and the edges are lightly browned.
6. Allow to cool before serving these addictive Kale Chips with Parmesan.

Nutritional Information (per serving):
- Calories: 120
- Protein: 4g
- Carbohydrates: 10g
- Fat: 7g
- Fiber: 3g

Stuffed Grape Leaves with Quinoa and Herbs

Delight your taste buds with Stuffed Grape Leaves with Quinoa and Herbs. These Mediterranean-inspired delights are filled with a savory mixture of quinoa and herbs, creating a flavorful side or snack that's both satisfying and nutritious.

Total Time: 50 minutes
Servings: 6

Ingredients:
- 1 jar grape leaves in brine, drained and rinsed
- 1 cup quinoa, cooked
- 1/4 cup fresh dill, chopped
- 1/4 cup fresh mint, chopped
- 1/4 cup pine nuts, toasted
- 2 tablespoons olive oil
- 1 lemon, juiced
- Salt and pepper to taste

Directions:
1. In a bowl, combine cooked quinoa, chopped dill, chopped mint, toasted pine nuts, olive oil, lemon juice, salt, and pepper.
2. Lay out a grape leaf and place a small spoonful of the quinoa mixture in the center.
3. Fold the sides of the grape leaf over the filling and roll tightly.
4. Repeat with the remaining grape leaves and filling.
5. Serve these delectable Stuffed Grape Leaves with Quinoa and Herbs chilled or at room temperature.

Nutritional Information (per serving):
- Calories: 220
- Protein: 5g
- Carbohydrates: 30g
- Fat: 9g
- Fiber: 4g

Baked Sweet Potato Fries

Enjoy a healthier twist on a classic with Baked Sweet Potato Fries. These crispy fries are seasoned to perfection and baked to a golden brown, offering a delightful and nutritious alternative to traditional potato fries.

Total Time: 30 minutes
Servings: 4

Ingredients:
- 2 large sweet potatoes, cut into fries
- 2 tablespoons olive oil
- 1 teaspoon paprika

- 1/2 teaspoon garlic powder
- 1/2 teaspoon cumin
- Salt and pepper to taste

Directions:
1. Preheat the oven to 425°F (220°C).
2. In a bowl, toss sweet potato fries with olive oil, paprika, garlic powder, cumin, salt, and pepper.
3. Spread fries in a single layer on a baking sheet.
4. Bake in the preheated oven for 25-30 minutes or until fries are crispy and golden.
5. Allow to cool slightly before serving these delicious Baked Sweet Potato Fries.

Nutritional Information (per serving):
- Calories: 180
- Protein: 2g
- Carbohydrates: 30g
- Fat: 6g
- Fiber: 5g

Guacamole with Veggie Sticks

Dive into the creamy goodness of Guacamole with Veggie Sticks. This classic dip pairs perfectly with an assortment of colorful vegetable sticks, creating a refreshing and nutritious snack that's not only tasty but also loaded with essential vitamins and minerals.

Total Time: 15 minutes
Servings: 4

Ingredients:
- 3 ripe avocados, mashed
- 1 tomato, diced
- 1/4 cup red onion, finely chopped
- 1/4 cup cilantro, chopped
- 1 lime, juiced
- Salt and pepper to taste
- Assorted vegetable sticks (carrots, cucumber, bell peppers) for dipping

Directions:

1. In a bowl, combine mashed avocados, diced tomato, chopped red onion, chopped cilantro, lime juice, salt, and pepper.
2. Mix well until ingredients are evenly incorporated.
3. Serve the guacamole with an assortment of vegetable sticks for a delightful and healthy snacking experience.

Nutritional Information (per serving, guacamole only):

- Calories: 200
- Protein: 3g
- Carbohydrates: 15g
- Fat: 17g
- Fiber: 9g

Greek Yogurt and Herb Dip

Elevate your snack game with Greek Yogurt and Herb Dip. This creamy and flavorful dip combines the richness of Greek yogurt with a medley of herbs, creating a delicious and wholesome accompaniment for vegetable sticks, crackers, or pita bread.

Total Time: 15 minutes
Servings: 6

Ingredients:

- 1 cup Greek yogurt
- 2 tablespoons fresh dill, chopped
- 2 tablespoons fresh mint, chopped
- 1 tablespoon fresh parsley, chopped
- 1 clove garlic, minced
- 1 tablespoon lemon juice
- Salt and pepper to taste

Directions:

1. In a bowl, combine Greek yogurt, chopped dill, chopped mint, chopped parsley, minced garlic, lemon juice, salt, and pepper.
2. Mix well until the herbs are evenly distributed.
3. Chill the dip in the refrigerator for at least 30 minutes before serving this delightful Greek Yogurt and Herb Dip.

Nutritional Information (per serving):
- Calories: 60
- Protein: 5g
- Carbohydrates: 3g
- Fat: 3g
- Fiber: 0g

Quinoa and Black Bean Stuffed Mushrooms

Impress your guests with Quinoa and Black Bean Stuffed Mushrooms. These savory bites are filled with a protein-packed mixture of quinoa and black beans, creating a satisfying and flavorful side or snack that's both nutritious and delicious.

Total Time: 30 minutes
Servings: 4

Ingredients:
- 12 large mushrooms, stems removed and reserved
- 1/2 cup quinoa, cooked
- 1/2 cup black beans, canned and drained
- 1/4 cup red onion, finely chopped
- 1/4 cup cherry tomatoes, diced
- 1/4 cup feta cheese, crumbled
- 1 tablespoon olive oil
- 1 teaspoon cumin
- Salt and pepper to taste

Directions:
1. Preheat the oven to 375°F (190°C).
2. Finely chop the reserved mushroom stems.
3. In a pan, sauté chopped mushroom stems, red onion, and olive oil until softened.
4. In a bowl, combine cooked quinoa, black beans, sautéed mushroom mixture, diced cherry tomatoes, crumbled feta cheese, cumin, salt, and pepper.
5. Stuff each mushroom cap with the quinoa and black bean mixture.
6. Bake in the preheated oven for 15-20 minutes or until mushrooms are tender.
7. Serve these Quinoa and Black Bean Stuffed Mushrooms warm.

Nutritional Information (per serving):
- Calories: 180
- Protein: 8g

- Carbohydrates: 20g
- Fat: 8g
- Fiber: 4g

Deviled Eggs with Hummus

Put a twist on a classic with Deviled Eggs with Hummus. These creamy and flavorful deviled eggs are filled with a luscious hummus mixture, creating a unique and protein-rich snack that's perfect for any gathering.

Total Time: 20 minutes
Servings: 6

Ingredients:
- 6 hard-boiled eggs, peeled and halved
- 1/4 cup hummus
- 1 tablespoon Greek yogurt
- 1 teaspoon Dijon mustard
- 1 tablespoon fresh chives, chopped
- Paprika for garnish
- Salt and pepper to taste

Directions:
1. Remove the yolks from the halved hard-boiled eggs and place them in a bowl.
2. Mash the egg yolks and mix with hummus, Greek yogurt, Dijon mustard, chopped chives, salt, and pepper.
3. Spoon the hummus mixture back into the egg whites.
4. Sprinkle it with paprika for garnish.
5. Chill before serving these Deviled Eggs with Hummus.

Nutritional Information (per serving):
- Calories: 90
- Protein: 7g
- Carbohydrates: 2g
- Fat: 6g
- Fiber: 1g

Zucchini Fritters with Greek Yogurt Sauce

Enjoy a crispy and flavorful treat with Zucchini Fritters with Greek Yogurt Sauce. These golden fritters are made with shredded zucchini and a blend of herbs, served with a cooling Greek yogurt sauce for a delightful side or snack.

Total Time: 35 minutes
Servings: 4

Ingredients:
For the Zucchini Fritters:
- 2 medium zucchinis, grated
- 1/2 cup feta cheese, crumbled
- 1/4 cup fresh dill, chopped
- 1/4 cup fresh parsley, chopped
- 1/4 cup green onions, chopped
- 1/4 cup all-purpose flour
- 1 egg, beaten
- 1 teaspoon baking powder
- Salt and pepper to taste
- Olive oil for frying

For the Greek Yogurt Sauce:
- 1/2 cup Greek yogurt
- 1 tablespoon lemon juice
- 1 tablespoon fresh mint, chopped
- Salt and pepper to taste

Directions:
For the Zucchini Fritters:
1. Place grated zucchini in a clean kitchen towel and squeeze out excess moisture.
2. In a bowl, combine grated zucchini, crumbled feta cheese, chopped dill, chopped parsley, chopped green onions, all-purpose flour, beaten egg, baking powder, salt, and pepper.
3. Heat olive oil in a pan over medium heat.
4. Drop spoonfuls of the zucchini mixture into the pan and flatten into fritters.
5. Cook for 3-4 minutes on each side or until golden brown.
6. Drain on paper towels.

For the Greek Yogurt Sauce:
1. In a bowl, combine Greek yogurt, lemon juice, chopped mint, salt, and pepper.
2. Mix well.

Serve the Zucchini Fritters with a side of Greek Yogurt Sauce.

- Calories: 220
- Protein: 8g
- Carbohydrates: 15g
- Fat: 15g
- Fiber: 2g

Almond and Herb-Crusted Cauliflower Bites

Indulge in the crispy goodness of Almond and Herb-Crusted Cauliflower Bites. These bite-sized delights are coated in a flavorful almond and herb mixture, baked to perfection, and served with a zesty dipping sauce for a satisfying and wholesome side or snack.

Total Time: 45 minutes
Servings: 4

Ingredients:
For the Almond and Herb-Crusted Cauliflower:
- 1 head cauliflower, cut into florets
- 1 cup almonds, finely ground
- 1/4 cup fresh parsley, chopped
- 2 tablespoons nutritional yeast
- 1 teaspoon garlic powder
- 1 teaspoon dried thyme
- 1/2 teaspoon paprika
- Salt and pepper to taste
- 2 eggs, beaten

For the Zesty Dipping Sauce:
- 1/2 cup Greek yogurt
- 1 tablespoon Dijon mustard
- 1 tablespoon lemon juice
- 1 teaspoon honey
- Salt and pepper to taste

Directions:
For the Almond and Herb-Crusted Cauliflower:
1. Preheat the oven to 400°F (200°C).
2. In a bowl, combine finely ground almonds, chopped parsley, nutritional yeast, garlic powder, dried thyme, paprika, salt, and pepper.

3. Dip each cauliflower floret into the beaten eggs and then coat with the almond and herb mixture.
4. Place coated cauliflower on a baking sheet lined with parchment paper.
5. Bake in the preheated oven for 25-30 minutes or until cauliflower is golden and crispy.

For the Zesty Dipping Sauce:
1. In a bowl, combine Greek yogurt, Dijon mustard, lemon juice, honey, salt, and pepper.
2. Mix well.

Serve the Almond and Herb-Crusted Cauliflower Bites with the Zesty Dipping Sauce.

Nutritional Information (per serving):
- Calories: 230
- Protein: 12g
- Carbohydrates: 18g
- Fat: 14g
- Fiber: 6g

Dessert

Berry and Almond Crisp

Indulge in the perfect balance of sweetness and crunch with Berry and Almond Crisp. This delightful dessert combines a medley of fresh berries with a nutty almond topping, creating a comforting and satisfying treat that's both wholesome and delicious.

Total Time: 40 minutes
Servings: 6

Ingredients:
For the Berry Filling:
- 4 cups mixed berries (strawberries, blueberries, raspberries, blackberries)
- 1/4 cup granulated sugar
- 1 tablespoon lemon juice
- 1 tablespoon cornstarch

For the Almond Crisp Topping:
- 1 cup rolled oats
- 1/2 cup almond flour
- 1/4 cup chopped almonds
- 1/4 cup maple syrup
- 2 tablespoons coconut oil, melted
- 1 teaspoon vanilla extract
- Pinch of salt

Directions:
For the Berry Filling:
1. Preheat the oven to 350°F (175°C).
2. In a bowl, combine mixed berries, granulated sugar, lemon juice, and cornstarch.
3. Transfer the berry mixture to a baking dish.

For the Almond Crisp Topping:
1. In a separate bowl, combine rolled oats, almond flour, chopped almonds, maple syrup, melted coconut oil, vanilla extract, and a pinch of salt.
2. Sprinkle the almond crisp topping evenly over the berries.
3. Bake in the preheated oven for 25-30 minutes or until the berries are bubbling, and the topping is golden brown.

Nutritional Information (per serving):
- Calories: 280

- Protein: 6g
- Carbohydrates: 40g
- Fat: 12g
- Fiber: 6g

Chocolate Avocado Mousse

Satisfy your sweet cravings with a healthier twist on chocolate mousse – Chocolate Avocado Mousse. This velvety and rich dessert combines the creaminess of ripe avocados with the decadence of dark chocolate, creating a guilt-free indulgence that's both delicious and nourishing.

Total Time: 15 minutes
Servings: 4

Ingredients:
- 2 ripe avocados
- 1/2 cup unsweetened cocoa powder
- 1/2 cup maple syrup
- 1 teaspoon vanilla extract
- Pinch of salt
- Fresh berries for garnish (optional)

Directions:
1. In a blender or food processor, combine ripe avocados, cocoa powder, maple syrup, vanilla extract, and a pinch of salt.
2. Blend until smooth and creamy.
3. Spoon the Chocolate Avocado Mousse into serving glasses.
4. Chill in the refrigerator for at least 1 hour before serving.
5. Garnish with fresh berries if desired.

Nutritional Information (per serving):
- Calories: 220
- Protein: 3g
- Carbohydrates: 30g
- Fat: 12g
- Fiber: 7g

Baked Apples with Cinnamon and Walnuts

Enjoy the comforting aroma of cinnamon and the natural sweetness of baked apples with this wholesome dessert – Baked Apples with Cinnamon and Walnuts. This simple and nutritious treat is a delightful way to satisfy your sweet tooth.

Total Time: 45 minutes
Servings: 4

Ingredients:
- 4 medium apples, cored and halved
- 2 tablespoons melted coconut oil
- 2 tablespoons maple syrup
- 1 teaspoon ground cinnamon
- 1/4 cup chopped walnuts

Directions:
1. Preheat the oven to 375°F (190°C).
2. In a bowl, toss cored and halved apples with melted coconut oil, maple syrup, and ground cinnamon.
3. Place the apples in a baking dish, cut side up.
4. Sprinkle chopped walnuts over the apples.
5. Bake in the preheated oven for 30-35 minutes or until the apples are tender.
6. Serve these Baked Apples warm, optionally with a dollop of Greek yogurt.

Nutritional Information (per serving):
- Calories: 180
- Protein: 2g
- Carbohydrates: 25g
- Fat: 9g
- Fiber: 5g

Coconut Chia Pudding

Treat yourself to a delightful and nutrient-packed dessert with Coconut Chia Pudding. This creamy and satisfying pudding combines the goodness of chia seeds with the tropical flavor of coconut, creating a sweet and wholesome treat.

Total Time: 4 hours (includes chilling time)
Servings: 4

Ingredients:
- 1/2 cup chia seeds
- 2 cups coconut milk
- 1/4 cup maple syrup
- 1 teaspoon vanilla extract
- Shredded coconut for garnish

Directions:
1. In a bowl, whisk together chia seeds, coconut milk, maple syrup, and vanilla extract.
2. Cover the bowl and refrigerate for at least 4 hours or overnight, allowing the chia seeds to absorb the liquid and form a pudding-like consistency.
3. Before serving, stir the Coconut Chia Pudding to ensure an even texture.
4. Spoon into serving glasses and garnish with shredded coconut.
5. Enjoy this Coconut Chia Pudding chilled.

Nutritional Information (per serving):
- Calories: 220
- Protein: 4g
- Carbohydrates: 20g
- Fat: 14g
- Fiber: 8g

Greek Yogurt Parfait with Honey and Pistachios

Delight your senses with the layers of flavor and texture in this Greek Yogurt Parfait with Honey and Pistachios. This elegant and nutritious dessert features creamy Greek yogurt, drizzled with honey, and topped with crunchy pistachios for a perfect balance of sweetness and crunch.

Total Time: 10 minutes
Servings: 2

Ingredients:
- 2 cups Greek yogurt
- 4 tablespoons honey
- 1/4 cup pistachios, chopped
- Fresh mint leaves for garnish (optional)

Directions:

1. In serving glasses, layer Greek yogurt, drizzle with honey, and sprinkle chopped pistachios.
2. Repeat the layers until the glasses are filled.
3. Finish with a drizzle of honey and a garnish of fresh mint leaves if desired.
4. Serve this Greek Yogurt Parfait with Honey and Pistachios chilled.

Nutritional Information (per serving):

- Calories: 320
- Protein: 18g
- Carbohydrates: 40g
- Fat: 12g
- Fiber: 2g

Pumpkin Pie Smoothie Bowl

Indulge in the flavors of fall with a healthy twist in the Pumpkin Pie Smoothie Bowl. This delightful dessert alternative brings together the seasonal goodness of pumpkin with a creamy texture, providing a satisfying treat that's as nutritious as it is delicious.

Total Time: 10 minutes
Servings: 2

Ingredients:

- 1 cup canned pumpkin puree
- 1 frozen banana
- 1/2 cup Greek yogurt
- 1/2 cup almond milk
- 1 teaspoon pumpkin pie spice
- 1 tablespoon maple syrup (optional)
- Toppings: Granola, sliced almonds, pumpkin seeds, and a drizzle of honey

Directions:

1. In a blender, combine pumpkin puree, frozen banana, Greek yogurt, almond milk, pumpkin pie spice, and maple syrup (if using).
2. Blend until smooth and creamy.
3. Pour the smoothie into bowls.
4. Top with granola, sliced almonds, pumpkin seeds, and a drizzle of honey.
5. Enjoy this Pumpkin Pie Smoothie Bowl immediately.

Nutritional Information (per serving):
- Calories: 250
- Protein: 10g
- Carbohydrates: 40g
- Fat: 5g
- Fiber: 8g

Poached Pears in Red Wine

Elevate your dessert experience with the sophisticated and elegant Poached Pears in Red Wine. This classic dessert combines the sweetness of pears with the rich flavors of red wine and warm spices, creating a luxurious treat that's perfect for special occasions.

Total Time: 45 minutes
Servings: 4

Ingredients:
- 4 ripe but firm pears, peeled and cored
- 2 cups red wine
- 1/2 cup granulated sugar
- 1 cinnamon stick
- 3 cloves
- 1 orange peel (strips)
- Vanilla ice cream for serving (optional)

Directions:
1. In a saucepan, combine red wine, granulated sugar, cinnamon stick, cloves, and orange peel.
2. Bring the mixture to a simmer over medium heat.
3. Add peeled and cored pears to the simmering red wine mixture.
4. Simmer for 25-30 minutes or until the pears are tender but still firm.
5. Remove the pears from the poaching liquid and let them cool slightly.
6. Serve the Poached Pears in Red Wine on a plate, drizzled with some of the poaching liquid.
7. Optionally, serve with a scoop of vanilla ice cream for added indulgence.

Nutritional Information (per serving, without ice cream):
- Calories: 180
- Protein: 1g
- Carbohydrates: 45g

- Fat: 0g
- Fiber: 4g

Banana Almond Bites

Enjoy a simple and wholesome sweet treat with Banana Almond Bites. These bite-sized delights combine the natural sweetness of bananas with the nutty crunch of almonds, creating a snack that's not only delicious but also packed with nutrients.

Total Time: 20 minutes
Servings: 4

Ingredients:
- 2 ripe bananas, mashed
- 1/2 cup almond flour
- 1/4 cup almond butter
- 1 teaspoon vanilla extract
- Pinch of salt
- 1/4 cup dark chocolate chips (optional, for drizzling)

Directions:
1. In a bowl, combine mashed bananas, almond flour, almond butter, vanilla extract, and a pinch of salt.
2. Mix until well combined.
3. Scoop tablespoon-sized portions of the mixture and roll them into bite-sized balls.
4. Place the Banana Almond Bites on a parchment-lined tray.
5. Optionally, melt dark chocolate and drizzle it over the bites for added sweetness.
6. Chill in the refrigerator for at least 10 minutes before serving.

Nutritional Information (per serving):
- Calories: 180
- Protein: 4g
- Carbohydrates: 20g
- Fat: 10g
- Fiber: 3g

Dark Chocolate Covered Strawberries

Indulge in a classic and romantic dessert with Dark Chocolate Covered Strawberries. This simple yet elegant treat pairs the natural sweetness of ripe strawberries with the rich and decadent flavor of dark chocolate, creating a delightful and guilt-free dessert.

Total Time: 20 minutes
Servings: 6

Ingredients:
- 1 pint fresh strawberries, washed and dried
- 4 ounces dark chocolate, chopped
- 1 tablespoon coconut oil
- Chopped nuts or shredded coconut for garnish (optional)

Directions:
1. In a heatproof bowl, melt dark chocolate and coconut oil over a double boiler or in the microwave in 30-second intervals, stirring until smooth.
2. Dip each strawberry into the melted chocolate, coating it halfway.
3. Place the chocolate-covered strawberries on a parchment-lined tray.
4. Optionally, sprinkle chopped nuts or shredded coconut over the chocolate while it's still wet.
5. Chill in the refrigerator for at least 10 minutes to allow the chocolate to set.
6. Serve these Dark Chocolate Covered Strawberries at room temperature.

Nutritional Information (per serving):
- Calories: 120
- Protein: 2g
- Carbohydrates: 15g
- Fat: 7g
- Fiber: 3g

Mango Sorbet with Mint

Cool down and refresh your palate with the tropical delight of Mango Sorbet with Mint. This fruity and minty dessert is a perfect way to enjoy the vibrant flavors of mango while staying light and refreshing.

Total Time: 4 hours (includes freezing time)
Servings: 4

Ingredients:
- 3 cups frozen mango chunks
- 1/4 cup fresh mint leaves
- 1/4 cup honey or maple syrup
- 1 tablespoon lime juice
- Mint leaves for garnish (optional)

Directions:
1. In a blender, combine frozen mango chunks, fresh mint leaves, honey or maple syrup, and lime juice.
2. Blend until smooth and creamy.
3. Transfer the mixture to a shallow dish and spread it evenly.
4. Freeze for at least 4 hours or until the Mango Sorbet is firm.
5. Before serving, let the sorbet sit at room temperature for a few minutes to soften slightly.
6. Scoop into bowls, garnish with mint leaves if desired, and enjoy this Mango Sorbet with Mint.

Nutritional Information (per serving):
- Calories: 120
- Protein: 1g
- Carbohydrates: 30g
- Fat: 0g

Smoothies

Green Detox Smoothie with Kale and Pineapple

Kickstart your day with a burst of freshness and nourishment in the Green Detox Smoothie with Kale and Pineapple. Packed with nutrient-rich kale and the tropical sweetness of pineapple, this smoothie is a vibrant and invigorating way to support your body's natural detoxification process.

Total Time: 10 minutes
Servings: 2

Ingredients:
- 2 cups fresh kale, stems removed
- 1 cup pineapple chunks
- 1 banana
- 1/2 cucumber, peeled
- 1 tablespoon chia seeds
- 1 cup coconut water
- Ice cubes (optional)

Directions:
1. In a blender, combine fresh kale, pineapple chunks, banana, peeled cucumber, chia seeds, and coconut water.
2. Blend until smooth and creamy.
3. Add ice cubes if a colder consistency is desired.
4. Pour the Green Detox Smoothie into glasses and enjoy this revitalizing start to your day.

Nutritional Information (per serving):
- Calories: 150
- Protein: 5g
- Carbohydrates: 35g
- Fat: 2g
- Fiber: 8g

Berry Blast Smoothie with Flaxseeds

Energize your body and satisfy your taste buds with the Berry Blast Smoothie with Flaxseeds. This vibrant and antioxidant-rich smoothie combines a medley of berries with the omega-3 goodness of flaxseeds, creating a delicious and nutritious blend that's perfect for a quick and healthy snack.

Total Time: 8 minutes
Servings: 2

Ingredients:
- 1 cup mixed berries (strawberries, blueberries, raspberries)
- 1/2 cup plain Greek yogurt
- 1 tablespoon flaxseeds
- 1 tablespoon honey
- 1 cup almond milk
- Ice cubes (optional)

Directions:
1. In a blender, combine mixed berries, plain Greek yogurt, flaxseeds, honey, and almond milk.
2. Blend until smooth and creamy.
3. Add ice cubes if desired for a colder consistency.
4. Pour the Berry Blast Smoothie into glasses and enjoy the burst of berry goodness.

Nutritional Information (per serving):
- Calories: 180
- Protein: 8g
- Carbohydrates: 25g
- Fat: 6g
- Fiber: 7g

Tropical Turmeric Smoothie

Transport yourself to a tropical paradise with the Tropical Turmeric Smoothie. This vibrant and anti-inflammatory blend combines the exotic flavors of pineapple and mango with the golden touch of turmeric, creating a delicious and health-boosting smoothie to brighten your day.

Total Time: 12 minutes
Servings: 2

Ingredients:
- 1 cup mango chunks
- 1 cup pineapple chunks
- 1 banana
- 1/2 teaspoon turmeric powder
- 1 tablespoon fresh ginger, grated
- 1 tablespoon chia seeds
- 1 cup coconut water
- Ice cubes (optional)

Directions:
1. In a blender, combine mango chunks, pineapple chunks, banana, turmeric powder, grated ginger, chia seeds, and coconut water.
2. Blend until smooth and creamy.
3. Add ice cubes if a colder consistency is preferred.
4. Pour the Tropical Turmeric Smoothie into glasses and savor the tropical goodness.

Nutritional Information (per serving):
- Calories: 170
- Protein: 4g
- Carbohydrates: 40g
- Fat: 2g
- Fiber: 8g

Spinach and Banana Smoothie

Boost your energy levels and nourish your body with the vibrant Spinach and Banana Smoothie. Packed with nutrient-dense spinach and the natural sweetness of banana, this smoothie is a quick and delicious way to incorporate more greens into your diet.

Total Time: 8 minutes
Servings: 2

Ingredients:
- 2 cups fresh spinach
- 2 bananas
- 1/2 cup plain Greek yogurt
- 1 tablespoon almond butter
- 1 cup almond milk
- Ice cubes (optional)

Directions:

1. In a blender, combine fresh spinach, bananas, plain Greek yogurt, almond butter, and almond milk.
2. Blend until smooth and creamy.
3. Add ice cubes if desired for a refreshing chill.
4. Pour the Spinach and Banana Smoothie into glasses and enjoy the nutrient-packed goodness.

Nutritional Information (per serving):

- Calories: 220
- Protein: 8g
- Carbohydrates: 35g
- Fat: 7g
- Fiber: 6g

Blueberry and Almond Milk Smoothie

Indulge in the rich and antioxidant-packed Blueberry and Almond Milk Smoothie. This smoothie combines the sweet-tart flavor of blueberries with the creamy goodness of almond milk, creating a delightful and nutrient-dense drink that's perfect for breakfast or a refreshing snack.

Total Time: 10 minutes
Servings: 2

Ingredients:

- 1 cup blueberries (fresh or frozen)
- 1 banana
- 1/2 cup plain almond milk
- 1/4 cup rolled oats
- 1 tablespoon almond butter
- 1 teaspoon honey
- Ice cubes (optional)

Directions:

1. In a blender, combine blueberries, banana, almond milk, rolled oats, almond butter, and honey.
2. Blend until smooth and creamy.
3. Add ice cubes if a colder consistency is desired.

4. Pour the Blueberry and Almond Milk Smoothie into glasses and relish the delicious blend of flavors.

Nutritional Information (per serving):
- Calories: 200
- Protein: 5g
- Carbohydrates: 35g
- Fat: 6g
- Fiber: 7g

Avocado and Spinach Smoothie

Experience a creamy and nutrient-packed delight with the Avocado and Spinach Smoothie. This green powerhouse combines the richness of avocado with the vibrant freshness of spinach, creating a smoothie that's not only delicious but also loaded with essential vitamins and minerals.

Total Time: 8 minutes
Servings: 2

Ingredients:
- 1 ripe avocado, peeled and pitted
- 2 cups fresh spinach
- 1 banana
- 1/2 cup Greek yogurt
- 1 tablespoon chia seeds
- 1 cup almond milk
- Ice cubes (optional)

Directions:
1. In a blender, combine ripe avocado, fresh spinach, banana, Greek yogurt, chia seeds, and almond milk.
2. Blend until smooth and creamy.
3. Add ice cubes if desired for a refreshing chill.
4. Pour the Avocado and Spinach Smoothie into glasses and revel in the creamy goodness.

Nutritional Information (per serving):
- Calories: 250
- Protein: 8g

- Carbohydrates: 30g
- Fat: 14g
- Fiber: 9g

Cucumber and Mint Smoothie

Refresh your senses with the hydrating and invigorating Cucumber and Mint Smoothie. This light and crisp smoothie combines the cooling properties of cucumber with the aromatic freshness of mint, creating a perfect beverage to quench your thirst and revitalize your day.

Total Time: 6 minutes
Servings: 2

Ingredients:
- 1 cucumber, peeled and chopped
- 1 cup fresh mint leaves
- 1 green apple, cored and chopped
- 1 tablespoon lime juice
- 1 tablespoon honey
- 1 cup coconut water
- Ice cubes (optional)

Directions:
1. In a blender, combine chopped cucumber, fresh mint leaves, chopped green apple, lime juice, honey, and coconut water.
2. Blend until smooth and refreshing.
3. Add ice cubes if a colder consistency is preferred.
4. Pour the Cucumber and Mint Smoothie into glasses and savor the revitalizing taste.

Nutritional Information (per serving):
- Calories: 120
- Protein: 2g
- Carbohydrates: 30g
- Fat: 1g
- Fiber: 6g

Kiwi and Kale Smoothie

Boost your immune system and enjoy a burst of vitamins with the Kiwi and Kale Smoothie. This vibrant green blend combines the tropical sweetness of kiwi with the nutrient-dense goodness of kale, creating a delicious and health-enhancing smoothie.

Total Time: 8 minutes
Servings: 2

Ingredients:
- 2 kiwis, peeled and sliced
- 2 cups fresh kale, stems removed
- 1 banana
- 1/2 cup plain Greek yogurt
- 1 tablespoon chia seeds
- 1 cup water or coconut water
- Ice cubes (optional)

Directions:
1. In a blender, combine sliced kiwis, fresh kale, banana, plain Greek yogurt, chia seeds, and water or coconut water.
2. Blend until smooth and vibrant.
3. Add ice cubes if a colder consistency is desired.
4. Pour the Kiwi and Kale Smoothie into glasses and relish the tropical goodness.

Nutritional Information (per serving):
- Calories: 180
- Protein: 6g
- Carbohydrates: 35g
- Fat: 3g
- Fiber: 10g

Pineapple Coconut Smoothie

Transport yourself to a tropical paradise with the luscious Pineapple Coconut Smoothie. This exotic blend combines the sweetness of pineapple with the creamy goodness of coconut, creating a refreshing and indulgent smoothie that's perfect for a quick getaway from the everyday.

Total Time: 6 minutes
Servings: 2

Ingredients:
- 2 cups pineapple chunks
- 1/2 cup coconut milk
- 1 banana
- 1/2 cup plain Greek yogurt
- 1 tablespoon shredded coconut
- Ice cubes (optional)

Directions:
1. In a blender, combine pineapple chunks, coconut milk, banana, plain Greek yogurt, and shredded coconut.
2. Blend until smooth and tropical.
3. Add ice cubes if a colder consistency is preferred.
4. Pour the Pineapple Coconut Smoothie into glasses and enjoy the taste of paradise.

Nutritional Information (per serving):
- Calories: 220
- Protein: 6g
- Carbohydrates: 40g
- Fat: 8g
- Fiber: 5g

Orange and Carrot Smoothie

Start your day with a burst of vitamin C and beta-carotene in the Orange and Carrot Smoothie. This zesty and vibrant blend combines the citrusy goodness of oranges with the earthy sweetness of carrots, creating a refreshing and immune-boosting smoothie.

Total Time: 8 minutes
Servings: 2

Ingredients:
- 3 oranges, peeled and segmented
- 1 cup carrots, peeled and chopped
- 1 banana
- 1/2 cup plain Greek yogurt
- 1 tablespoon honey
- 1 cup water or orange juice
- Ice cubes (optional)

Directions:

1. In a blender, combine orange segments, chopped carrots, banana, plain Greek yogurt, honey, and water or orange juice.
2. Blend until smooth and citrusy.
3. Add ice cubes if a colder consistency is desired.
4. Pour the Orange and Carrot Smoothie into glasses and revel in the vitamin-packed goodness.

Nutritional Information (per serving):

- Calories: 190
- Protein: 6g
- Carbohydrates: 40g
- Fat: 1g
- Fiber: 7g

"Whenever you find yourself doubting how far you can go, just remember how far you have come. Remember everything you have faced, all battles you have won, and all fears you have overcome."

Conclusion

As we reach the conclusion of the "Diverticulitis Diet Cookbook," let's take a moment to reflect on the journey we've embarked on together—a journey toward better health, well-being, and a lifestyle that supports the management of diverticulitis. Throughout this cookbook, we've explored not only the delicious recipes designed specifically for individuals dealing with diverticulitis but also the fundamental principles of a diverticulitis-friendly diet.

One of the primary lessons we've learned is the transformative power of mindful eating. Understanding diverticulitis and its dietary impact has allowed us to make informed choices about the foods we consume, empowering us to take control of our health. The importance of a specialized diverticulitis diet has been emphasized, highlighting the role of specific nutrients and dietary adjustments in managing symptoms and promoting overall well-being.

The foundations of a diverticulitis-friendly diet have been laid out, emphasizing the incorporation of high-fiber foods, lean proteins, and gut-friendly ingredients. We've explored not only what to include in our meals but also what to avoid, creating a roadmap for a diet that supports digestive health.

As we conclude this cookbook, it's essential to recognize the positive changes that can result from conscious choices and intentional dietary habits. Remember, the journey to better health is not a sprint but a marathon, and each small step contributes to a healthier, more vibrant future.

To everyone who has embarked on this journey, whether you are managing diverticulitis or simply seeking a diet that promotes digestive wellness, commend yourself for your commitment to your health. The patient's success story shared in the introduction serves as a testament to the real impact that practical strategies and dietary changes can have on one's life.

In the pursuit of long-term wellness, don't forget the significance of lifestyle changes. Beyond the kitchen, incorporating habits such as regular physical activity, stress management, and adequate hydration contributes to a holistic approach to well-being.

As you continue to explore the recipes and embrace the principles outlined in this cookbook, let it be a starting point for a healthier, more vibrant life. Every recipe you try, every meal you savor, and every choice you make brings you closer to a future where digestive health is a cornerstone of your overall well-being.

Thank you for joining us on this culinary and wellness journey. Here's to your health, to mindful eating, and to a future filled with vitality and balance. May these recipes and insights serve as companions on your ongoing quest for a life well-lived and enjoyed to the fullest. Cheers to a healthier, happier you!